Clinical Case Studies for the

Nutrition Care Process

Elizabeth Zorzanello Emery, MS, RD, CNSC, LDN

Assistant Professor
Nutrition Program
La Salle University
School of Nursing and Health Sciences
Philadelphia, Pennsylvania

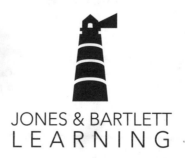

JONES & BARTLETT
LEARNING

World Headquarters

Jones & Bartlett Learning	Jones & Bartlett Learning	Jones & Bartlett Learning
5 Wall Street	Canada	International
Burlington, MA 01803	6339 Ormindale Way	Barb House, Barb Mews
978-443-5000	Mississauga, Ontario L5V 1J2	London W6 7PA
info@jblearning.com	Canada	United Kingdom
www.jblearning.com		

Jones & Bartlett Learning books and products are available through most bookstores and online book-sellers. To contact Jones & Bartlett Learning directly, call 800-832-0034, fax 978-443-8000, or visit our website, www.jblearning.com.

Substantial discounts on bulk quantities of Jones & Bartlett Learning publications are available to corporations, professional associations, and other qualified organizations. For details and specific discount information, contact the special sales department at Jones & Bartlett Learning via the above contact information or send an email to specialsales@jblearning.com.

The cases in this book are based on the clinical experiences of the author and contributors, and were designed for educational purposes. Resemblance to individual patients should be considered coincidental.

The author, editor, and publisher have made every effort to provide accurate information. However, they are not responsible for errors, omissions, or for any outcomes related to the use of the contents of this book and take no responsibility for the use of the products and procedures described. Treatments and side effects described in this book may not be applicable to all people; likewise, some people may require a dose or experience a side effect that is not described herein. Drugs and medical devices are discussed that may have limited availability controlled by the Food and Drug Administration (FDA) for use only in a research study or clinical trial. Research, clinical practice, and government regulations often change the accepted standard in this field. When consideration is being given to use of any drug in the clinical setting, the health care provider or reader is responsible for determining FDA status of the drug, reading the package insert, and reviewing prescribing information for the most up-to-date recommendations on dose, precautions, and contraindications, and determining the appropriate usage for the product. This is especially important in the case of drugs that are new or seldom used.

Production Credits

Publisher, Higher Education: Cathleen Sether
Senior Acquisitions Editor: Shoshanna Goldberg
Senior Associate Editor: Amy L. Bloom
Editorial Assistant: Prima Bartlett
Associate Marketing Manager: Jody Sullivan
Production Director: Amy Rose
Senior Production Editor: Renée Sekerak
Production Assistant: Sean Coombs
V.P., Manufacturing and Inventory Control: Therese Connell
Photo Researcher: Lian Bruno
Cover Design: Scott Moden
Composition: Laserwords Private Limited, Chennai, India
Printing and Binding: Malloy, Inc.
Cover Printing: Malloy, Inc.

Library of Congress Cataloging-in-Publication Data
Emery, Elizabeth Zorzanello.
  Clinical case studies for the nutrition care process / Elizabeth Zorzanello Emery.
    p. ; cm.
  Includes bibliographical references.
  ISBN-13: 978-0-7637-6184-4 (pbk.)
  ISBN-10: 0-7637-6184-2 (pbk.)
  1. Diet therapy—Case studies. 2. Nutrition—Case studies. I. Title.
  [DNLM: 1. Nutrition Therapy—Case Reports. 2. Dietary Services—Case Reports. 3. Nutritional Physiological Phenomena—Case Reports. WB 400]
  RM216.E524 2012
  615.8′54—dc23
                                                    2011025144

6048
Printed in the United States of America
15 14 13 12 11   10 9 8 7 6 5 4 3 2 1

To my father, Joe Zorzanello, who together with my beloved mother, Margaret, taught me that with faith and determination, anything is possible.

Contents

Preface

I have had the great privilege of working with many talented professionals, courageous patients, and inquisitive students in my years of dietetics practice. One of the things that inspired me to write this book was the positive response that I got from students whenever I brought credible cases into my classroom. Students were actually asking for additional case studies to complete, and commenting on the value of case-based learning years after graduation. With the introduction of standardized terminology and the Nutrition Care Process, I began to see that students and seasoned professionals alike needed a way to apply this new paradigm to the traditional practice of medical nutrition therapy. This book intends to give realistic scenarios for a variety of cases organized in the format of the Nutrition Care Process. It is intended to be used along with a good medical nutrition therapy textbook and the ADA's *International Dietetics and Nutrition Terminology Reference Manual*. The cases have all been classroom tested. The answers have been extensively researched and referenced, and are available securely online for instructors and clinical managers, so students are stimulated to research, think critically, use evidence-based guidelines, and formulate their own answers to the questions. In many instances there is no single correct answer to a question, and your clinical judgment or new evidence may add another twist to the case. I hope that you will find these cases to be a valuable supplement to your classroom or staff development agenda.

Acknowledgments

I would like to thank my dean, Dr. Zane Wolf, for encouraging me to write this book; my colleagues Jule Anne Henstenberg, Susan Adams, and Eileen Chopnick for working alongside of me during the process; all of my talented contributors for their time and expertise; my sister, Mary Zorzanello, MSN, APRN, CNN, for reviewing the hemodialysis case; my editors, Shoshanna Goldberg and Amy Bloom, for their patience and encouragement; Valerie Bradley for administrative support; my students who critically tested the case studies, especially Danielle DiMarco, who also prepared the appendix on enteral formulas; and my children, Elisabeth, Marissa, and Nicholas, for their love and support.

Lastly, I'd like to express my appreciation to the following reviewers, whose feedback helped shape the text: Prithiva Chanmugam, PhD, RD, LDN, Louisiana State University; Amy Strickland, MS, RD, University of North Carolina at Greensboro; Joseph C. Bonilla, PhD, RD, University of the Incarnate Word; and Mallory Boylan, PhD, RD, LD, Texas Tech University.

Contributors

Susan E. Adams, MS, RD, LDN
Case 4, **Cultural Awareness**
Assistant Professor, Nutrition Program
La Salle University
School of Nursing and Health Sciences
Philadelphia, PA

Rodney D. Bell, MD, FAHA
Case 9, **Hypertension in a Middle-Aged Man**
Professor of Neurology and Neurosurgery
Vice Chairman Department of Neurology for Hospital Affairs
Chief Division of Cerebrovascular Disease and Neuro-critical Care
Thomas Jefferson Medical College
Philadelphia, PA

Stephen M. Clarke, MS, RD, LDN, CNSD
Case 21, **Nutrition Support for Burns**
Clinical Dietitian Specialist
Temple University Hospital
Philadelphia, PA

Sharon Del Bono, RD, CNSD, LDN
Case 20, **Nutrition Support of the Critically Ill Trauma Patient**
Nutrition Support Dietitian, Surgical ICU
Temple University Hospital
Philadelphia, PA

Debra DeMille, MS, RD, CSO
Case 16, **Pancreatic Cancer Status Post-Whipple Procedure**
Nutrition Counselor
Joan Karnell Cancer Center at Pennsylvania Hospital
Philadelphia, PA

Angela Grassi, MS, RD, LDN
Case 14, **Polycystic Ovary Syndrome in a Young Woman**
Director, PCOS Nutrition Center
Haverford, PA

Jule Anne D. Henstenberg, MS, RD, CSP, LDN
Case 7, **Childhood Obesity**
Director, Didactic Program in Nutrition and
  Coordinated Program in Dietetics
La Salle University
School of Nursing and Health Sciences
Philadelphia, PA

Bethany Jung, MS, RD, CNSC
Case 6, **Food Allergies in a Toddler**
Neonatal Dietitian
Newark Beth Israel Medical Center
Newark, NJ

Lisa M. Laura, RD, JD
Case 10, **Heart Failure in an Obese Woman**
Instructor, Nutrition Program
La Salle University
School of Nursing and Health Sciences
Philadelphia, PA

Rosanne Leibhart, MS, RD, CNSC, LDN
Case 10, **Heart Failure in an Obese Woman**
Assistant Director, Patient Services
Underwood-Memorial Hospital
Woodbury, NJ

Cheryl Marco, RD, CDE, LDN
Case 12, **Advanced Dietary Management in Type 1 Diabetes**
Registered Dietitian/Certified Diabetes Educator
Division of Endocrinology, Diabetes & Metabolic Diseases
Thomas Jefferson University
Philadelphia, PA

Jodi Horwitz Nehila, MS, RD, LDN
Case 5, **Failure to Thrive in Infancy**
Coordinator of Nutrition Services
Weisman Children's Rehabilitation Hospital
Marlton, NJ

Dana O'Connell, MA, RD, LDN
Case 18, **HIV/AIDS with Wasting**
Outpatient/HIV Dietitian
Albert Einstein Medical Center
Philadelphia, PA

Abhijit S. Pathak, MD, FACS
Case 20, **Nutrition Support of the Critically Ill Trauma Patient**
Professor of Surgery
Temple University School of Medicine
Director, Surgical ICU
Temple University Hospital
Philadelphia, PA

Steven R. Peikin, MD, FACG, AGAF
Case 19, **Exacerbation of Crohn's Disease**
Head, Division of Gastroenterology and Liver Diseases
Cooper University Hospital
Professor of Medicine, Robert Wood Johnson Medical School
Camden, NJ

Marianna Siokos, RD, LDN
Case 15, **Chronic Kidney Disease: Nutrition for Hemodialysis**
Renal Dietitian
Fresenius Medical Care
Philadelphia, PA

Introduction

BACKGROUND

What did you *do* for the patient? Why should you be paid for your services? Can you show that you actually helped? These are a few of the many provocative questions that bear a real significance in today's healthcare world. With an aging population and rising rates of chronic conditions such as obesity, diabetes, cardiovascular disease, and cancer, healthcare expenditures continue to spiral. Shrinking healthcare reimbursements are looming in the face of uncertainties regarding healthcare reform. Assuring that care is appropriate, timely, and cost effective is critical in today's healthcare environment.

A shift to evidence-based practice and the use of electronic health records (EHR) are two trends that have emerged from the need to assure quality of health care while controlling costs. Evidence-based practice involves using the best available research to support clinical decision making, and evolved in part due to recognized variations in clinical practice that occur when relying on limited clinical experience (1). Expert developers of evidence-based guidelines scour the literature and grade the strength of the evidence found to make recommendations that support practice. Evidence-based practice and electronic health records are intended to make care more consistent and improve communication between caregivers.

The federal push to create and use EHR by the year 2014 was spurred by the need to improve the safety and efficiency of health care (2). Safety, efficiency, quality, access, cost control, and research are all components of the government initiative to improve health care through the use of EHRs. Inherent to the use of EHRs is a standardized vocabulary set that can be utilized to track similar problems, interventions, and outcomes. Many professions already use standardized language, such as International Classification of Diseases (ICD) or Current Procedural Terminology (CPT) codes and Systematized Nomenclature of Medicine (SNOMED) (3,4). In 2003, the American Dietetic Association introduced its Nutrition Care Process and Model, which for the first time included a nutrition diagnosis that would be expressed using standardized terminology (5). It also set the stage for developing outcomes research to assess the effectiveness of nutrition care and to support evidence-based nutrition.

THE NUTRITION CARE PROCESS AND MODEL

The Nutrition Care Process and Model (NCPM) is a problem-solving method intended to optimize nutrition-related outcomes and enhance the recognition of registered dietitians (RDs) and dietetic technicians (DTRs) as preferred providers of nutrition services (6,7). It involves four steps at its core: nutrition assessment, diagnosis, intervention, and monitoring/evaluation. Nutrition screening and referral may feed into the process, but are separate from it, as these functions are not necessarily performed by nutrition professionals. Likewise, data from the Nutrition Care Process are funneled into an outcomes management system for aggregate evaluation of outcomes, a task that is not unique to RDs and DTRs. The four core steps of the process are considered to be functions that are the sole responsibilities of RDs and DTRs.

Nutrition Assessment

Nutrition assessment is a systematic approach for gathering and interpreting data that help to identify nutrition-related problems (6,8–10). It is an ongoing process of evaluation and reevaluation of pertinent indicators compared to accepted criteria. The nutrition assessment terms are grouped into 5 categories: food/nutrition-related history; anthropometric measurements; biochemical data, medical tests, and procedures; nutrition-focused physical findings; and client history (Table I–1) (8).

The RD determines the relevant data to analyze and assesses whether there is a need for additional information. The data are compared to an individualized goal or a reference standard chosen by the RD, such as a weight-based nutrient calculation versus the Recommended Dietary Allowance (RDA) for that nutrient. Based on the findings of the nutrition assessment, a nutrition-related problem or problems may be identified. These are then labeled as a nutrition diagnosis.

Table I–1 Nutrition Assessment Parameters (8)

Category	Examples
Food/Nutrition-related history	Food and nutrient intake, usual diet, medications, food availability, knowledge/beliefs about food, physical activity level.
Anthropometric measurements	Height, weight, body mass index, growth velocity, circumferences, etc.
Biochemical data, medical tests, and procedures	Lab data such as electrolytes, glucose, lipids; tests such as resting metabolic rate, abdominal X-rays, etc.
Nutrition-focused physical findings	Skin turgor and integrity, dentition, appearance of subcutaneous fat/muscle mass, etc.
Client History	Medical/surgical/family history, social history.

Nutrition Diagnosis

The nutrition diagnosis is a nutrition-related problem that nutrition professionals are responsible for treating (6,10). It is different from a medical diagnosis in that it is expected to resolve or improve through nutrition intervention. For example, a patient with stage 5 chronic kidney disease (CKD) on hemodialysis could have a nutrition diagnosis of excessive fluid intake, which would be evident from inappropriate interdialytic weight gains and edema. The edema and weight gain could be ameliorated by a fluid restriction, but the underlying medical problem of CKD would remain.

The nutrition diagnosis is written as a *problem*, *etiology*, *signs*/symptoms (PES) statement (8) (Table I–2). The "problem" is chosen from the list of standardized terms, which includes 70 diagnostic terms covering the following three domains: food and/or nutrient intake, clinical, and behavioral/environmental problems (7). The etiology is considered to be the underlying cause of the nutrition problem. It is a factor gathered during the assessment that contributes to the imbalance or difficulty noted. It follows the nutrition diagnostic term by the words "related to," for instance, excessive fluid intake related to food and nutrition-related knowledge deficit. In this example, it is assumed that the patient is unaware of the proper amount of fluid to consume, a factor that would have been identified during the assessment. The final part of the PES statement is the signs and symptoms, which are stated after the words "as evidenced by." In this example, the PES statement might read, excessive fluid intake related to

Table I–2 The PES Statement (8)

Problem	related to	Etiology	as evidenced by	Signs and Symptoms
Choose from one of 70 diagnostic terms		Factors identified in assessment; intervention is aimed here		Measurable assessment parameters that are monitored and evaluated for improvement

food and nutrition-related knowledge deficit as evidenced by 10 pound weight gain between dialysis treatments (8). The signs and symptoms are considered to be evidence (or proof) that the nutrition diagnosis exists. These should be stated in measurable terms, so that they can be monitored to assess progress toward goals at a predetermined assessment interval.

The PES statement should focus on the most pressing problem. The clinician may choose more than one nutrition diagnosis and write a PES statement for each. These should be prioritized and treated according to a plan that is acceptable to the patient or healthcare team. The statements should be clear and concise, include a single problem, relate to one etiology, and be based on documented assessment data (6). The PES statement links the assessment with the next step, intervention.

Nutrition Intervention

The nutrition intervention is a planned action intended to resolve the etiology of the nutrition problem or relieve the signs and symptoms noted in the PES statement (Table I–3) (8,10). It consists of two phases: planning and implementation. Now that you have identified a problem and determined its cause, what are you going to do and how are you going to do it? How can you close the gap between what the patient is currently taking in and how they would ideally be nourished? What type of diet or nutritional support do you recommend for the patient, and how will you execute your plan? The intervention is aimed at the etiology of the problem, and is intended to positively change factors contributing to the problem. When possible it should be substantiated by published evidence-based guidelines from the American Dietetic Association (ADA) or other professional organizations, evidence libraries such as the ADA's Evidence Analysis Library (EAL) or the Cochrane database, or current research or outcome studies (6,10).

Table I–3 Nutrition Intervention

Category	Types of Intervention
Food and/or nutrient delivery	Oral diets, enteral and parenteral nutrition, supplements, feeding assistance, feeding environment, nutrition-related medication management.
Nutrition education	Basic education on content and survival skills.
Nutrition counseling	Theoretical, cognitive, behavior-based counseling for self efficacy and self management.
Coordination of nutrition care	Team meetings, referral to experts or outside agencies.

The intervention should be planned and prioritized based on importance and feasibility. It should then be implemented in collaboration with the patient or client and the healthcare team. Goals of intervention should be communicated, along with time and frequency of follow-up care. The intervention can then be modified as needed depending on the patient or client's response. There are 90 terms to categorize specific interventions in the following four domains: 1) food and/or nutrient delivery, 2) nutrition education, 3) nutrition counseling, and 4) coordination of nutrition care (7). Included in these domains are oral diets, enteral and parenteral nutrition, supplements, feeding assistance, feeding environment, nutrition-related medication management, nutrition education, nutrition counseling, and coordination of care both during and after active treatment (8). Use of these terms will ultimately help in tracking the outcomes of our interventions.

Monitoring and Evaluation

The last step is monitoring and evaluation (6,8). This procedure helps to measure progress toward goals and whether or not problems have improved or resolved. It also helps to illuminate the results, or outcomes, of our treatments. The first step in monitoring is verifying implementation of the plan (6). Does the patient understand the diet? Is the prescribed enteral formula running at the optimal rate? Is the supplement being accepted and tolerated? The second step is to measure outcomes. Based on indicators identified in your assessment, measure any changes. Are the signs and symptoms improving? Lastly, evaluate outcomes, or results of your treatment. Compare present conditions with previous findings, established goals, and/or reference standards. If there is variance from expected results, investigate the reasons for the discrepancy. The nutrition intervention should be modified as needed to move toward goals. If the signs and symptoms have improved sufficiently, the nutrition diagnosis may be deemed to be resolved, and the patient can be monitored for a change in status or reevaluated for new problems.

Monitoring and evaluation terms have been combined with assessment terms, since the two are so closely related. There are over 300 assessment terms, with nearly 250 of them also used for monitoring and evaluation (7, 8). The assessment terms that relate to client history are used for assessment only, because they do not change as a result of intervention (8). Monitoring and evaluation terms fall under the categories of food/nutrition-related history; anthropometric measurements; biochemical data, medical tests, and procedures; and nutrition-focused physical findings (8). Monitoring and evaluation will help to track outcomes related to specific nutrition diagnoses, interventions, and goals. The use of standardized monitoring and evaluation terms facilitates data collection and improves the strength of the findings. Overall, the four steps of the nutrition care process and model help us to be consistent with practice guidelines published by the ADA.

STANDARDS OF PRACTICE (SOP)

The ADA's Standards of Practice (SOP), Standards of Professional Performance (SOPP), and Code of Ethics serve to guide the practice and performance of RDs and DTRs in all settings (11). The SOPs are composed of four principles representing the four steps of the Nutrition Care Process. The standards are designed to promote safety, efficacy, and efficiency in the practice of evidence-based food and nutrition services, and result in improved outcomes (11). In addition, the standards are intended to encourage continuous quality improvement, research, innovation, and professional development of RDs. The standards specify that RDs use pertinent data to identify nutrition-related problems, label specific nutrition problems that they are responsible for treating, plan and implement interventions, monitor progress, and evaluate outcomes (11). The Standards of Practice thus direct us to use the Nutrition Care Process in order to be in compliance with the scope of practice for our profession (12).

HOW DOES IT ALL FIT TOGETHER?

The Nutrition Care Process combines the art and science of nutrition care. A skilled diagnostician can combine clinical judgment with astute observation powers and evidence driven decisions to deliver the best care, in the most cost-effective manner, communicated in a way that can be universally understood and tracked. The Nutrition Care Process is supported by the Standards of Professional Practice, the Evidence Analysis Library, and standardized language (Figure I–1).

It is incumbent on us as professionals to provide the best care that we can, and to show that it works at the same time. We are expected by accreditors and consumers alike to follow the standards of practice that our profession has set out for us, which include using the Nutrition Care Process. Embracing this process will help us to identify and describe comparable nutrition-related problems, treatments, and results, thereby expanding evidence-based research and practice in the field of nutrition. It also facilitates the inclusion of unique nutrition services into electronic health records, which will help our profession to move forward as the nation adopts new health informatics technology.

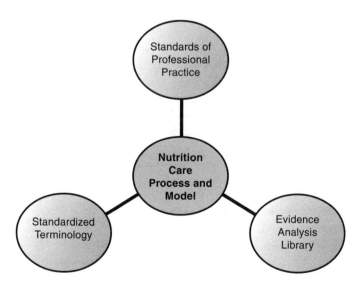

Figure I–1. The Nutrition Care Process is supported by the Standards of Professional Practice, the Evidence Analysis Library, and standardized language.

REFERENCES

1. Gray GE, Gray LK. Evidence-based medicine: applications in dietetic practice. *J Am Diet Assoc.* 2002; 102:1263–1272.
2. Hoggle LB, Michael MA, Houston SM, Ayers EJ. Electronic health record: where does nutrition fit in? *J Am Diet Assoc.* 2006; 106:1688–1695.
3. Hakel-Smith N, Lewis NM. A Standardized nutrition care process and language are essential components of a conceptual model to guide and document nutrition care and patient outcomes. *J Am Diet Assoc.* 2004; 104:1878–1884.
4. Atkins M, Basualdo-Hammond C, Hotson B. Canadian perspectives on the nutrition care process and International Dietetics and Nutrition terminology. *Can J Diet Pract Res.* 2010; 71:e18–e20.
5. Lacey K, Pritchett E. Nutrition care process and model: ADA adopts road map to quality care and outcomes management. *J Am Diet Assoc.* 2003; 103:1061–1072.
6. Nutrition care process and model part I: the 2008 update. *J Am Diet Assoc.* 2008; 108:1113–1117.
7. Nutrition care process part II: using the International Dietetics and Nutrition Terminology to document the nutrition care process. *J Am Diet Assoc.* 2008; 108:1287–1293.
8. American Dietetic Association (ADA): *International Dietetics & Nutrition Terminology (IDNT) Reference Manual: Standardized Language for the Nutrition Care Process*, 3rd ed. Chicago, IL: American Dietetic Association; 2011.
9. Charney P. The nutrition care process and the nutrition support dietitian. *Support Line.* 2007; 29:4, 18–22.
10. Skipper A. Applying the nutrition care process: nutrition diagnosis and intervention. *Support Line.* 2007; 29:6, 12–23.
11. American Dietetic Association Revised 2008 Standards of Practice for Registered Dietitians in Nutrition Care; Standards of Professional Performance for Registered Dietitians; Standards of Practice for Dietetic Technicians, Registered, in Nutrition Care; and Standards of Professional Performance for Dietetic Technicians, Registered. *J Am Diet Assoc.* 2008; 108:1538-1542.
12. Gardner-Cardani J, Yonkoski D, Kerestes J. Nutrition care process implementation: a change management perspective. *J Am Diet Assoc.* 2007; 107: 1429–1433.

PART

I

General Nutrition Care

General Nutritional Assessment

LEARNING OBJECTIVES

Upon completing this case study, readers will be able to:

1. Recognize anthropometric, biochemical, clinical, and dietary factors that impact on nutritional status.
2. Calculate and interpret weight change and body mass index.
3. Determine adequacy of dietary intake.
4. Apply the Nutrition Care Process to an elderly patient.

CASE DESCRIPTION/BACKGROUND

Adequate nutrition can be viewed as a state of balance between intake, requirements, metabolism, and losses of nutrients. The term *malnutrition* usually refers to a state of undernutrition, and has been associated with increased morbidity and mortality in the clinical setting (1–4). The accurate identification of patients at risk for malnutrition and its associated complications is both an art and a science; subjective and objective data are interpreted along with clinical judgment to evaluate nutritional status.

From the dietary standpoint, a full evaluation considers not only calorie and protein intake but also vitamin and mineral status.

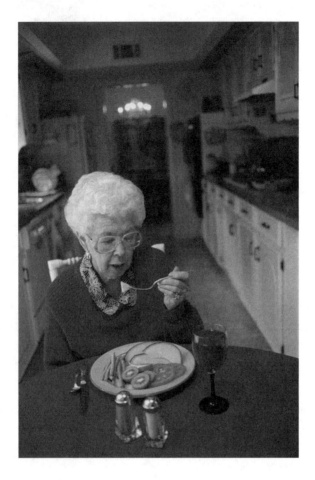

Surrogate markers of visceral protein stores such as serum albumin and prealbumin have traditionally been measured for nutritional assessment. These parameters are now known to be affected by many factors, including hydration, physiological stress, and inflammation. Particularly during metabolic stress, serum proteins more specifically reflect severity of illness than nutritional stores (1–7). While a low serum albumin is associated with increased morbidity and mortality, it cannot be used alone to measure nutritional status or repletion. Conversely, a normal serum albumin cannot be used in isolation to rule out malnutrition. Serum protein levels by themselves do not form the basis for nutrition diagnosis or intervention. Individual assessment parameters should be considered as part of a bigger picture of nutritional equilibrium.

The client is a 76-year-old woman with a history of hypertension admitted to the hospital after tripping over her cat and falling at home. She is admitted for a femur fracture. She is currently confined to bed.

NUTRITIONAL ASSESSMENT DATA

1. Anthropometric Measurements.

Height: 67″
Weight: 140 lbs
Usual weight: 160 lbs 6 months ago. She has been unmotivated to cook since the loss of her husband during the previous 6 months.

2. Biochemical Data, Medical Tests, and Procedures.

a. Labs

Parameter	Value	Normal Range* (may vary by age, sex, and lab)
Sodium	140 mEq/L	135–147 mEq/L
Potassium	3.2 mEq/L	3.5–5.0 mEq/L
Chloride	103 mEq/L	98–106 mEq/L
Carbon dioxide	29 mEq/L	21–30 mEq/L
BUN	19 mg/dL	8–23 mg/dL
Creatinine	1.0 mg/dL	0.7–1.5 mg/dL
Glucose	108 mg/dL	70–110 mg/dL
Hemoglobin	12.0 g/dL	12–16 g/dL (female)
Hematocrit	38.1 %	36–47 % (female)
Albumin	3.2 g/dL	3.5–5.5 g/dL
Prealbumin	11 mg/dL	16–40 mg/dL

*Data from U. S. Food and Drug Administration. *Investigations Operations Manual.* Silver Spring, MD: US FDA; 2001. Accessed April 12, 2011 from http://www.fda.gov/downloads/ICECI/Inspections/IOM/UCM135835.pdf

Morris JC. *Dietitian's Guide to Assessment and Documentation.* Sudbury, MA: Jones & Bartlett Learning; 2011.

b. Test results, if pertinent

X-ray indicates fracture of left femoral neck.

3. Nutrition-Focused Physical Findings.

Blood pressure: 128/65 mm Hg

Oral mucosa dry. Has upper and lower dentures which are poorly fitting.

Skin turgor decreased.

4. Client History.

Social Hx

No smoking or alcohol

Husband died 6 months ago and patient has lost weight since that time

Family Hx

N/A

5. Food/Nutrition-Related History.

Usual Diet

Breakfast

1 cup (8 oz) decaffeinated tea with 1 tbs half and half and 1 tsp sugar

1 slice white toast with 1 tsp margarine and 1 tsp jelly or 1 frozen pancake with 1 tbs syrup

½ cup orange juice

Lunch

Canned soup, usually chicken noodle, 1 cup

4 unsalted crackers with 2 tbs peanut butter

½ cup sliced peaches in light syrup

Sweetened iced tea, 1 cup

Dinner

Chicken thigh with skin, stewed

½ cup rice or potato with 1 tsp margarine

½ cup spinach or carrots
1 cup (8 oz) decaffeinated tea with 1 tbs cream and 1 tsp sugar

Notes

Rarely eats or drinks between meals.
Avoids eggs and milk due to food preferences.

Medications

Furosemide 20 mg daily

Supplements

None

QUESTIONS

1. Convert her height and weight to centimeters and kilograms. Calculate her % IBW, % UBW, and BMI. Interpret her weight and weight change based on these parameters.
2. Calculate her nutritional requirements (calories, protein, and fluid) and compare her current intake to her needs.
3. Are any major food groups and nutrients obviously missing from her diet? Explain your answer.
4. Do you think she could be experiencing any drug–nutrient interactions? If so, what dietary suggestions would you make?
5. Interpret her serum albumin and prealbumin. In addition to nutritional intake, what factors can cause these indices to drop? What factors would cause them to be elevated?
6. Describe how factors in her anthropometric, biochemical, clinical, and dietary nutritional assessment data all fit together to form a "picture" of her nutritional health.
7. Write a PES statement based on the nutritional assessment data available.
8. What dietary and social changes would you suggest to improve her nutritional intake?
9. What are your nutritional goals for her, and how would you monitor the effectiveness of your interventions from question #8?
10. Write a note documenting your assessment in the SOAP or ADIME format.

REFERENCES AND SUGGESTED READINGS

1. Barbosa-Silva M. Subjective and objective nutritional assessment methods: what do they really assess? *Curr Opin Clin Nutr Metab Care.* 2008; 11: 248–254.

2. Marshall WJ. Nutritional assessment: its role in the provision of nutritional support. *J Clin Pathol.* 2008; 61:1083–1088.

3. Hall JC: Nutritional Assessment of Surgery Patients. *J Am Coll Surg.* 2005; 202:5, 837–843.

4. Fuhrman MP. The albumin–nutrition connection: separating myth from fact. *Nutrition.* 2002; 18:199–200.

5. Delegge MH, Drake LM. Nutritional assessment. *Gastroenterol Clin N Am.* 2007; 36:1–22.

6. Fuhrman MP, Charney P, and Mueller CM. Hepatic proteins and nutrition assessment. *JADA.* 2004; 104:1258–1264.

7. Shenkin A. Serum prealbumin: is it a marker of nutritional status or of risk of malnutrition? *Clin Chem.* 2006; 52:12, 2177–2178.

8. Shah B, Sucher K, Hollenbeck C. Comparison of ideal body weight equations and published height-weight tables with body mass index tables for healthy adults in the United States. *Nutr Clin Pract.* 2006; 21:312–319.

9. Jeejeebhoy K. Nutritional assessment. *Nutrition.* 2000; 16:7/8, 585–590.

10. U.S. Department of Agriculture (USDA), Agricultural Research Service. 2010. USDA National Nutrient Database for Standard Reference, Release 23. *Nutrient Data Laboratory Home Page.* Accessed April 12, 2011, from http://www.ars.usda.gov/nutrientdata

11. American Dietetic Association (ADA), *International Dietetics & Nutrition Terminology (IDNT) Reference Manual: Standardized Language for the Nutrition Care Process*, 3rd ed. Chicago, IL: ADA; 2010.

Drug–Nutrient Interactions

LEARNING OBJECTIVES

Upon completing this case study, readers will be able to:

1. Recognize the importance of food and medication interactions.
2. Explain the relationship between the anticoagulant warfarin and Vitamin K.
3. Identify food sources of Vitamin K.
4. Suggest dietary adjustments to avoid common food medication interactions.

CASE DESCRIPTION/BACKGROUND

Food and drug interactions can be both the cause and effect of altered absorption, metabolism, action, and excretion of involved drugs and nutrients (1). Herbal and dietary components can affect the potency of many medications, leading to increased toxicity or decreased effectiveness of the medications (2). Furthermore, medications can compromise nutritional status by impacting on the intake or absorption of nutrients. While there are many potential food and medication interactions, one of the more common potential problems exists between the anticoagulant warfarin and dietary Vitamin K. The Joint Commission's Hospital National Safety Goals specifically address the safety of anticoagulation therapy, and stipulate that education is given on food and drug interactions for patients receiving warfarin (3).

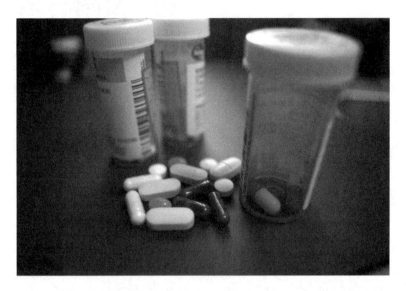

Anticoagulation therapy is used in conditions such as atrial fibrillation, deep vein thrombosis, pulmonary embolus, prosthetic heart valves, and hypercoagulable states (4). Warfarin is a common oral anticoagulant that acts as a Vitamin K antagonist, inhibiting several coagulation factors in the normal blood clotting process (4,5). Striking a balance between too little and too much anticoagulation is a major objective of therapy, because the therapeutic window is relatively narrow and risks of excessive bleeding can be significant (5). International normalized ratio (INR) is a relative measure of blood clotting time that is monitored closely during therapy; adjustments to both medications and diet may be made according to changing INR levels.

The patient is a 66-year-old woman with hypertension, hyperlipidemia, atrial fibrillation, and chronic urinary tract infections. She has a history of a mild subcortical stroke with no neurologic deficits. She is extremely fearful that a future stroke would leave her unable to care for herself. She lives with her husband and does most of the cooking; they follow a heart healthy diet. She has great difficulty maintaining a stable INR. The INR has been either too high or too low and her warfarin dose has been changed multiple times. She is referred by her cardiologist for dietary advice.

NUTRITIONAL ASSESSMENT DATA

1. Anthropometric Measurements.

Height: 5'5"
Weight: 131 lbs

2. Biochemical Data.

Parameter	Result	Normal Range* (may vary)
INR	4.0 seconds	2.0–3.0 seconds
Total cholesterol	189 mg/dL	< 200 mg/dL
LDL cholesterol	90 mg/dL	< 100 mg/dL with preexisting heart disease or diabetes < 130 mg/dL with heart disease risk factors
HDL cholesterol	44 mg/dL	> 40 mg/dL men > 50 mg/dL women
Triglyceride	100 mg/dL	< 150 mg/dL

*Data from American Heart Association. Third Report of the National Cholesterol Education Program (NCEP) Expert Panel on Detection, Evaluation, and Treatment of High Blood Cholesterol in Adults (Adult Treatment Panel III) final report. *Circulation* 2002; 106:3143. Hirsh J, Fuster V, Ansell J, Halperin JL. American Heart Association/American College of Cardiology Foundation guide to warfarin therapy. *Circulation* 2003; 107:1692–1711.

3. Nutrition-Focused Physical Findings.

The patient is an adequately nourished woman. She has multiple bruises on her extremities but denies any recent trauma. She complains of muscle aches.

Blood pressure: 136/75 mm Hg

4. Client History.

She does not drink or smoke. She is retired and lives with her husband.

5. Food/Nutrition-Related History.

Usual Diet

Breakfast

> cold cereal (fortified) or oatmeal
> grapefruit or orange juice
> wheat toast with butter
> coffee with milk

Lunch

> turkey sandwich on wheat bread with lettuce and tomato
> fresh or frozen berries with cottage cheese
> diet soda or tea

Afternoon snack

> piece of fruit
> mozzarella cheese stick
> wheat crackers

Dinner

> broiled chicken
> brown rice
> asparagus, spinach, or collard greens
> green salad with romaine lettuce and vinaigrette dressing
> fruit sorbet for dessert
> sparkling water, and a glass of wine once or twice weekly

Medications

> Simvistatin and warfarin. She takes bactrim periodically for urinary
> tract infections.

Supplements

> She had been taking St. John's wort for depression but recently
> stopped. She takes a multivitamin occasionally.

QUESTIONS

1. What is the Dietary Reference Intake (DRI) for Vitamin K? What is the Daily Value (DV) for Vitamin K as listed on food and supplement labels?
2. Identify sources of Vitamin K, both from diet and synthesis in the body.
3. Look up Vitamin K levels of the following sample foods in a food composition table or database: 1 cup of cooked kale, 1 cup turnip greens, 1 cup raw romaine lettuce, 1 cup raw peeled cucumber, 1 cup cooked turnips. How do the Vitamin K levels of these foods compare to the DRI and DV?
4. What is the recommended adjustment in Vitamin K intake in patients on warfarin? What foods should they avoid or limit?
5. Is it advisable for her to take a multivitamin? How much Vitamin K is in a standard "once daily" multivitamin?
6. How would her periodic use of antibiotics affect her INR?
7. Describe the effects of herbal supplements such as St. John's wort on medication.
8. Name other food medication interactions for which she is at risk.
9. Write a PES statement. What is your intervention?
10. How would you monitor and evaluate the results of your intervention?

REFERENCES AND SUGGESTED READINGS

1. Lingtak-Neader C. Drug-nutrient interaction in clinical nutrition. *Curr Opin Clin Nutr Metab Care*. 2002; 5:327–332.
2. Boullata J. Natural health products interaction with medication. *Nutr Clin Pract*. 2005; 20:33–51.
3. The Joint Commission Accreditation Program. National Patient Safety Goals. Accessed April 12, 2011, from http://www.jointcommission.org/standards_information/npsgs.aspx
4. Hirsh J, Fuster V, Ansell J, Halperin JL. American Heart Association/American College of Cardiology Foundation guide to warfarin therapy. *Circulation* 2003; 107:1692–1711.

5. Glasheen JJ. Preventing warfarin-related bleeding. *South Med J.* 2005; 98(1): 96–103.

6. United States Department of Agriculture (USDA), National Agriculture Library. *Dietary Guidance: Dietary Reference Intakes.* Accessed May 17, 2011 from http://fnic.nal.usda.gov/nal_display/index.php?info_center=4&tax_level=3&tax_subject=256&topic_id=1342&level3_id=5140

7. National Institutes of Health (NIH), Clinical Center. *Important information to know when you are taking: Coumadin and Vitamin K.* Bethesda, MD: NIH; 2003. Accessed April 12, 2011, from http://www.cc.nih.gov/ccc/patient_education/drug_nutrient/coumadin1.pdf

8. U.S. Department of Agriculture (USDA), Agricultural Research Service. 2010. USDA National Nutrient Database for Standard Reference, Release 23. *Welcome to the Nutrient Data Laboratory Home Page* (modified Dec 2010). Accessed April 12, 2011, from http://www.ars.usda.gov/nutrientdata

9. Penning-van Beest, FJ, van Meegen E, Rosendaal FR, Stricker BH. Drug interactions as a cause of overanticoagulation on phenprocoumon or acenocoumarol predominantly concern antibacterial drugs. *Clin Pharmacol Ther.* 2001; 69:451–457.

10. American Dietetic Association (ADA). *Pocket Guide for International Dietetics & Nutrition Terminology (IDNT) Reference Manual: Standardized Language for the Nutrition Care Process*, 3rd ed. Chicago, IL: ADA; 2010.

Osteoporosis in a Postmenopausal Woman

LEARNING OBJECTIVES

Upon completing this case study, readers will be able to:

1. Describe osteoporosis and osteopenia.
2. Identify risk factors for low bone density.
3. Apply basic nutritional and dietary assessment skills.
4. Differentiate between available forms of calcium supplements.
5. Suggest dietary interventions to optimize nutrient intake in a patient with osteoporosis.

CASE DESCRIPTION AND BACKGROUND

Osteoporosis is a debilitating disease that affects more than 10 million Americans (1,2). It is defined as low bone mass and deterioration of bone architecture that leads to structural fragility and increased risk for fractures, especially of the hip, spine, and wrist (1–4). It is estimated that by the year 2020, half of all Americans over age 50 will be at risk of an osteoporotic fracture (1,2). The results of these fractures can be devastating, leading to increased disability, morbidity, and mortality.

While many non-dietary factors contribute to the development of osteoporosis, proper nutrition plays a role in the prevention and treatment of this condition. Risk factors for postmenopausal osteoporosis include advanced age, genetic predisposition, low lifetime calcium and Vitamin D intake, smoking, excessive alcohol consumption, amenorrhea, use of certain medications, and thinness (BMI < 21 kg/m^2) (1–4). Calcium and Vitamin D are recommended in sufficient amounts to help prevent and treat osteoporosis (2). In addition, there is evidence that an overall dietary pattern that focuses on fruits and vegetables and avoids excessive protein and sodium chloride may help to promote bone health (5–8).

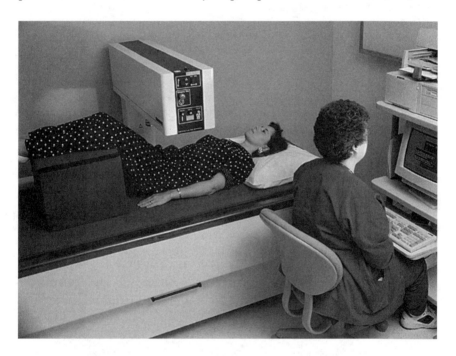

The client is a 55-year-old Caucasian secretary who completed menopause 5 years ago. She has had asthma since childhood and takes a steroid inhaler. She requires several courses of oral glucocorticoids during the winter, as she often has exacerbations of her asthma during the cold weather. One year ago, she was diagnosed with osteoporosis based on a Dexa Scan that indicated a T-score of –2.7 in the lumbar spine and –1.5 in the hips. She was started on alendronate sodium at that time.

She is now 4 weeks s/p right wrist fracture. She has been out of work because she cannot type. She is having trouble with normal activities of daily living due to her inability to use her dominant hand.

NUTRITIONAL ASSESSMENT DATA

1. Anthropometric Measurements.

Height: 5'4"
Weight: 117 lbs
Usual weight: 120 lbs

2. Biochemical Data.

Lab	Result	Normal Range* (may vary by age, sex, and lab)
Sodium	140 mEq/L	135–147 mEq/L
Potassium	4.1 mEq/L	3.5–5.0 mEq/L
Chloride	103 mEq/L	98–106 mEq/L
CO_2	24 mEq/L	21–30 mEq/L
BUN	11 mg/dL	8–23 mg/dL
Creatinine	0.7 mg/dL	0.7–1.5 mg/dL
Glucose	72 mg/dL	70–110 mg/dL
Albumin	3.2 mg/dL	3.5–5.5 g/dL
Calcium	8.3 mg/dL	8.5–10.8 mg/dL
25-OH Vitamin D_3	14 ng/mL	32–100 ng/mL

*Data from U. S. Food and Drug Administration (FDA). *Investigations Operations Manual.* Silver Spring, MD: US FDA; 2001. Accessed April 14, 2011, from http://www.fda.gov/downloads/ICECI/Inspections/IOM/UCM135835.pdf

Morris JC. *Dietitian's Guide to Assessment and Documentation.* Sudbury, MA: Jones & Bartlett Learning; 2011

Hollis B. Assessment and interpretation of circulating 25-hydroxyvitamin D and 1,25-dihydroxyvitamin D in the clinical environment. *Endocrinol Metab Clin N Am.* 2010; 39: 271–286.

3. Nutrition-Focused Physical Findings.

Right wrist immobilized in cast and sling.

4. Client History.

Social Hx

Does not smoke. Drinks socially.

5. Food/Nutrition-Related History.

Diet Hx

She has a history of lactose intolerance and reports avoiding many dairy products due to nausea and gas. She admits that she has never tried lactose-reduced milk and is unaware of alternate dietary sources of calcium. She reports that she doesn't enjoy cooking, so eats fast foods or dines out frequently. Since her wrist fracture, she has been eating mostly finger foods.

Typical intake:

Breakfast

bacon and egg breakfast sandwich
2 cups coffee with cream and sugar

Lunch

ham and American cheese sandwich on white bread
mustard 1 tsp
potato chips
water or diet cola

Dinner

fast food hamburger with a pickle spear
French fries with ketchup
iced tea

Snacks

Crackers and pretzels; drinks water during the day.

Medications

Alendronate sodium once weekly; Hx of glucocorticoid use.

Supplements

None

QUESTIONS

1. Define osteoporosis and osteopenia. What risk factors does she have for low bone density? Describe what a dual-energy X-ray absorptiometry (DXA) scan is, and what the resulting T-scores mean.

2. Does her serum calcium reflect total body calcium stores? Why or why not? Calculate her "corrected" serum calcium.

3. Explain how Vitamin D is produced in the body or obtained from food, and how it is subsequently activated in the body. What is the active form of Vitamin D?

4. What test is typically used to assess Vitamin D stores? Would it be helpful to measure the active metabolite identified in question #3? How does her Vitamin D level compare to expected levels, and how might that influence her bone status?

5. What are the suggested intakes of calcium and Vitamin D for an individual with osteoporosis according to the National Osteoporosis Foundation? How do these recommendations differ from the RDA? Does she meet her needs with diet?

6. How could she consume enough calcium and Vitamin D through foods, given her lactose intolerance? Evaluate her overall dietary pattern. In addition to getting more calcium in her diet, are there any other specific dietary or lifestyle changes (interventions) you would suggest?

7. How might her long-term use of glucocorticoids for asthma have contributed to her osteoporosis?

8. List commonly available forms of calcium and Vitamin D supplements and their recommended usage. Do you think this client might benefit from supplements, and if so, what would you recommend? What are the effects of excessive amounts of supplemental calcium and Vitamin D?

9. Write a PES statement for this client.

10. What are your overall nutritional goals for this client? What outcomes (results) would you monitor to be sure she is meeting her goals?

REFERENCES AND SUGGESTED READINGS

1. U.S. Department of Health and Human Services (DHHS). *Bone Health and Osteoporosis. A Report of the US Surgeon General.* Rockville, MD; 2004.

2. National Osteoporosis Foundation (NOF). *Clinician's Guide to Prevention and Treatment of Osteoporosis.* Washington, DC: National Osteoporosis Foundation; 2010.

3. World Health Organization (WHO) Scientific Group on the Prevention and Management of Osteoporosis. *Prevention and Management of Osteoporosis: Report of a WHO Scientific Group. (WHO technical report series; 921).* Geneva, Switzerland: World Health Organization; 2003.

4. Management of osteoporosis in postmenopausal women: 2010 position statement of The North American Menopause Society. *Menopause.* 2010; 17(1):25–54.

5. Fenton TR, Eliasziw AW, Tough SC, Hanley DA. Meta-analysis of the quantity of calcium excretion associated with the net acid excretion of the modern diet under the acid-ash diet hypothesis. *Am J Clin Nutr.* 2008; 88:1159–1166.

6. New SA. Intake of fruit and vegetables: implications for bone health. *Proc Nutr Soc.* 2003; 62:889–899.

7. Frassetto L, Morris RC Jr, Sellmeyer DE, Todd K, Sebastian A. Diet, evolution, and aging—the pathophysiologic effects of the post-agricultural inversion of the potassium-to-sodium and base-to-chloride ratios in the human diet. *Eur J Nutr.* 2001; 40:200–213.

8. Morgan SL. Nutrition and bone: it is more than calcium and vitamin D. *Women's Health.* 2009; 5(6):727–737.

9. Cherniak EP, Levis S, Troen BR. Hypovitaminosis D: a stealthy epidemic that requires treatment. *Geriatrics.* 2008; 63:4: 24–30.

10. Binkley N, Ramamurthy R, Krueger D. Low Vitamin D status: definition, prevalence, consequences, and correction. *Endocrinol Metab Clin N Am.* 2010; 39:287–301.

11. Hollis B. Assessment and interpretation of circulating 25-hydroxyvitamin D and 1,25-dihydroxyvitamin D in the clinical environment. *Endocrinol Metab Clin N Am.* 2010; 39:271–286.

12. Institute of Medicine (IOM). *Dietary Reference Intakes for Calcium and Vitamin D.* Washington, DC: National Academy of Sciences; released November 2010. Accessed April 14, 2011, from http://www.iom.edu/ Reports/2010/Dietary-Reference-Intakes-for-Calcium-and-Vitamin-D.aspx

13. Straub DS. Calcium supplementation in clinical practice: a review of forms, doses, and indications. *Nutr Clin Pract.* 2007; 22:286–296.

14. American Dietetic Association (ADA). *International Dietetics & Nutrition Terminology (IDNT) Reference Manual: Standardized Language for the Nutrition Care Process*, 3rd ed. Chicago, IL: American Dietetic Association; 2010.

Cultural Awareness

LEARNING OBJECTIVES

Upon completing this case study, readers will be able to:

1. Identify the unique cultural aspects (including specific cultural foods) that affect the client's nutritional health.
2. Assess the client's nutrition status based on the client's physical, medical, social, and diet history, and formulate a nutrition diagnosis based on the client's nutrition status.
3. Include the unique nutritional needs of older adults when developing a nutrition care plan for the age 65+ client.
4. Complete a nutrition screening of the client using a validated nutrition screening and assessment tool.
5. Develop a culturally-sensitive nutrition care plan for the client.

CASE DESCRIPTION/BACKGROUND

Cultural awareness and competence is an important skill that may challenge the dietetic student. These skills will become increasingly necessary as the demographic predictions are indicating that the U.S. population is becoming "larger, older, and more diverse" (1). By the year 2050, projected demographic shifts show that the black, Asian and Pacific Islander, American Indian, Eskimo and Aleut, and Hispanic-origin populations will increase their proportions of the total population while the non-Hispanic white population proportion will decrease (1). In addition, health disparities are well-documented to occur in some demographic groups including racial and ethnic minorities, women, children, elderly, residents of rural areas, and persons with disabilities (2).

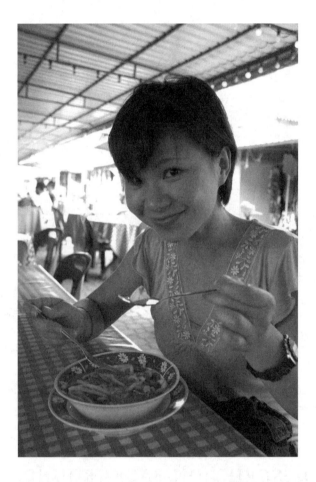

A January 2011 *Journal of the American Dietetic Association* report stated that a "dietary pattern consistent with current guidelines to consume relatively high amounts of vegetables, fruit, whole grains, poultry, fish, and low-fat dairy products may be associated with superior nutritional status, quality of life, and survival in older adults" (3). Clearly, successful aging can be promoted through increased understanding of the unique nutritional and cultural needs of older adults by the dietetic student and practitioner.

This case study involves a seemingly healthy Vietnamese woman who is being screened for an initial Medicare evaluation. Sixty-five years old is considered "young old" by the U.S. Census Bureau; however, this chronological age does not always indicate health status (4,5). Elderly individuals experience physiological changes associated with aging that may include concerns in oral health (chewing and swallowing), reduced appetite and thirst (with risk of subsequent dehydration), and age-related metabolic changes affecting the status of Vitamins D, B_{12}, and Vitamin A (5,6). The diets of elderly women need to be adequate in terms of energy to provide enough calories to cover the increased calcium needs of post-menopausal women.

A 65-year-old Vietnamese woman who has lived in an urban area of the United States for 35 years recently went to a primary care physician. She was responding to advice from her son to obtain the Initial Preventive Physical Examination (IPPE), which is standard procedure to starting enrollment in Medicare Services (7).

She speaks very little English but was able to converse with the physician through the services of a translator who was provided by the local Council on Aging (8). After the required elements of the IPPE (including past medical/surgical history, current medication and supplements, family history, history of alcohol, tobacco and illicit drug use, diet and physical activities as well as screening for depression, and a review of the individual's functional ability and level of safety), the physical examination was performed. This physical examination included the following: height, weight, blood pressure, a visual acuity screen, and determination of BMI (7).

In addition to the required elements of the examination, the attending physician completed the MNA Mini Nutritional Assessment—Short Form (MNA—SF), which is a validated tool for screening the elderly that is effective, inexpensive, quick, and easy to administer (9,10).

NUTRITIONAL ASSESSMENT DATA

1. Anthropometric Measurements.

Height: 59″
Weight: 95 lbs

2. Nutrition-Focused Physical Findings.

Patient appears of slight bone structure
Visual acuity screen: WNL
Dental health: partial upper dentures: oral health WNL
Blood pressure: 120/80 mm Hg

3. Client History.

Medical/surgical Hx

Not significant with only Caesarian section surgery (34 years ago).

Family Hx

She currently lives alone. Mother died recently at age 85 and suffered from "many bad bones." Father died in 1968 during the Vietnam War. American husband died two years ago of a heart attack. One son, age 34, lives out of the area with his wife and one child (boy) age 6.

4. Food/Nutrition-Related History.

Current Medications/Supplements

OTC aspirin for minor arthritis pain, ginseng for health, and hot ginger tea for indigestion.
24-Hour diet recall.

Breakfast

Congee with bits of shrimp or leftover pork, beef or chicken (total 1 cup)
green tea (plain without sugar) – usually 1 cup
perhaps some white toast spread with butter (1 slice with 1 tsp butter)

Lunch

pho (usually with beef) – 1 cup

small bowl of white rice – ¾ cup

small amount of fresh bean sprouts, lime wedges (2), and mint (a few
sprigs) in pho

green tea (plain without sugar) – one cup

small orange or ½ cup mango chunks

Mid-afternoon snack

mung beans (cooked and ground in water) ½ cup

ginger tea (plain without sugar)

Dinner

pho – leftover from lunch (one cup)

small bowl of white rice – ¾ cup

small amount of fresh bean sprouts, lime wedges (2), and mint in pho

spinach cooked in garlic and rendered chicken fat, and 1 tsp nuoc
mam sauce – (¾ cup)

green tea (plain without sugar) – (one cup)

small amount of mango chunks

When asked if her diet was typical, she indicated that she tries to eat
but has not been feeling well since "a bad wind made her cold" (cold and
flu symptoms), and thinks that she needs to eat more yang foods to
balance the illness. This is why on this particular day she elected to eat
mango, beef, and garlic because these are "yang" foods and will balance
her cold symptoms. The mung beans, she believes will help "even out" the
cold foods (11). The client states that she does not have much appetite
since her mother died two months ago and thinks she may have "lost
some weight because her clothes are loose now." She also tells the physician
that her nice neighbor has been bringing her pho for her meals.

Until the deaths of her husband and mother, she was a homemaker,
and also cooked and helped take care of her aging mother. Daily activities
included taking care of her home, grocery shopping, and the like. The
client is ambulatory and capable of all ADL. She denies alcohol and
tobacco use. Grocery shopping is accomplished by purchasing all food

from the corner store because she does not know how to drive a car. She depends on monthly social security payments and a small pension from her late husband, and may be eligible for the SNAP (Supplemental Nutrition Assistance Program) (6).

Note that in the Vietnamese culture, the patient would list their last name first, followed by their first name. When addressing this patient, the dietitian should call her "Miss" or "Mrs.", followed by her first name, as this is the custom in Vietnam (12).

QUESTIONS

1. Convert the client's height and weight to centimeters and kilograms. Calculate her % IBW, % UBW, and BMI. Review her BMI and interpret her weight and weight changes based on these parameters.
2. Access the Mini Nutritional Assessment–Short Form (MNA–SF) (http://www.mna-elderly.com/mna_forms.html) and complete the screening for this client. What is the MNA Score? Based on the MNA screening, what is your recommendation for future intervention?
3. Calculate her nutritional requirements (EER for calories and RDA or grams per kilogram for protein). List her requirements for fluid and fiber, as well as the RDA for Vitamins B_{12}, D, and A, and calcium.
4. Review her 24-hour dietary recall and calculate this day's calories, protein, carbohydrate, fat, fluid, fiber, and calcium levels. Are any food groups missing from her diet on this day? If this day's diet is typical, what nutrients might be low or missing from it?
5. Are there any red flags in the patient and diet histories that lead you to believe there might be a concern with her future nutritional health? Consider what is meant by her comment concerning her own ("a bad wind made her cold") and her mother's ("bad bones") health status.
6. Some of the foods consumed by this client might be unfamiliar to you. Describe the following foods.

   a. Pho
   b. Mung beans

    c. Congee

    d. Nuoc mam sauce

7. What are yang foods and "hot" and "cold" foods?

8. List two each alternative "yin" and "yang" foods that might be incorporated into her diet to help increase any nutritional deficiencies.

9. Write an appropriate nutrition diagnosis based on the available nutritional assessment data.

10. What are your nutritional goals for this client, based on her unique cultural background and nutrition diagnosis?

REFERENCES AND SUGGESTED READINGS

1. U.S. Census Bureau. *Population Profile of the United States.* Accessed April 15, 2011, from http://www.census.gov/population/www/pop-profile/natproj .html

2. Medline Plus, National Institute of Health (NIH). *Health Disparities.* Accessed April 15, 2011, from http://www.nlm.nih.gov/medlineplus/ healthdisparities.html

3. Anderson A, Harris TB, Tylaysky FA, et al. Dietary patterns and survival of older adults. *J Am Diet Assoc.* 2011; 111:84–91.

4. U.S. Census Bureau. *Current Population, Numerical Growth.* Accessed April 15, 2011, from http://www.census.gov/prod/1/pop/p23-190/p23190-f.pdf

5. Worthington-Roberts BS, Williams SR. *Nutrition Throughout the Life Cycle,* 4th ed. Boston, MA: McGraw-Hill; 2000.

6. Position Paper of the American Dietetic Association: Nutrition Across the Spectrum of Aging. *J Am Diet Assoc.* 2005; 105:616–633.

7. Medicare Preventive Services. *Quick Reference Information: The ABCs of Providing the Initial Preventive Physical Examination.* Accessed April 15, 2011, from https://www.cms.gov/MLNProducts/downloads/MPS_QRI_IPPE001a .pdf

8. McCaffree J. Language: a crucial part of cultural competency. *J Am Diet Assoc.* 2008; 108:611–613.

9. Nestle Nutrition Institute. MNA Mini Nutritional Assessment—Short Form (MNA—SF). Accessed April 15, 2011, from http://www.mna-elderly.com/ mna_forms.html

10. Tsai AC, Chang TL, Wang YC, Liao CY. Population-specific short-form Mini Nutritional Assessment with body mass index or calf circumference can predict risk of malnutrition in community-living or institutionalized elderly people in Taiwan. *J Am Diet Assoc.* 2010; 110:1328–1334.

11. Tu J. Nutrition and fasting in Vietnamese culture. Accessed April 15, 2011, from http://ethnomed.org/clinical/nutrition/viet-food/

12. Adopt Vietnam. Vietnamese names for girls. Accessed April 15, 2011, from http://www.adoptvietnam.org/vietnamese/names-girls.htm

13. Shah B, Sucher K, Hollenbeck C. Comparison of ideal body weight equations and published height-weight tables with body mass index tables for healthy adults in the United States. *Nutr Clin Pract.* 2006; 21(3): 312–319.

14. Institute of Medicine. *Dietary Reference Intakes Tables and Application.* Washington, DC: National Academy of Sciences. June 23, 2011. Accessed June 27, 2011 from http://www.iom.edu/Activities/Nutrition/SummaryDRIs/DRI-Tables.aspx

15. Kittler PG, Sucher KP. *Food and Culture*, 5th ed. Belmont, CA: Thompson Wadsworth; 2008.

16. Pennington AT, Douglass JS. *Bowes & Church's Food Values of Portions Commonly Used*, 18th ed. Philadelphia, PA: Lippincott Williams & Wilkins; 2005.

17. My Fitness Pal. *Search Vietnamese.* Accessed April 15, 2011, http://www.myfitnesspal.com/nutrition-facts-calories/vietnamese

18. Nguyen A. Viet world kitchen. Accessed April 15, 2011, from http://www.vietworldkitchen.com

19. Ohio State Extension. Fact Sheet. *Cultural Diversity: Eating in America.* Accessed April 15, 2011, from http://ohioline.osu.edu/hyg-fact/5000/pdf/5258.pdf

20. About.com. Yin and Yang in Chinese cooking. Accessed April 15, 2011, from http://chinesefood.about.com/library/weekly/aa101899.htm

21. USDA National Nutrient Database for Standard Reference. *Release 23, Vitamin D (D2 + D3).* Accessed April 15, 2011, from http://www.ars.usda.gov/SP2UserFiles/Place/12354500/Data/SR23/nutrlist/sr23a328.pdf

22. Gunther S, Patterson RE, Kristal AR, Stratton KL, White E. Demographic and health-related correlates of herbal and specialty supplement use. *J Am Diet Assoc.* 2004; 104:27–34.

23. American Dietetic Association (ADA). *International Dietetics & Nutrition Terminology (IDNT) Reference Manual: Standardized Language for the Nutrition Care Process*, 3rd ed. Chicago, IL: ADA; 2010.

Pediatrics

Failure to Thrive in Infancy

LEARNING OBJECTIVES

Upon completing this case study, readers will be able to:

1. Apply basic nutritional and dietary assessment skills for a special needs infant.
2. Identify causes of failure to thrive.
3. Calculate energy and protein needs for catch up growth.
4. Apply the nutrition care process to an infant with failure to thrive.

CASE DESCRIPTION/BACKGROUND

Failure to thrive (FTT) is a descriptive term applied to children whose growth is below the expected rate or measure. There can be many causes for FTT, including organic, nonorganic, and mixed causes. *Organic failure to thrive* includes medical conditions that prevent adequate intake, increase nutrient need, increase nutrient turnover, or increase energy expenditure. *Nonorganic failure to thrive* includes psychological and environmental factors that lead to inadequate intake. Many cases of failure to thrive involve multifactorial etiologies, such that a combination of organic and nonorganic factors contribute to growth failure (1). Although there is no single definition for FTT, it is generally recognized that the term applies to babies and children whose growth has been low or has decreased over time. Specific indicators include height or weight below the third to fifth percentiles on more than one occasion, or who fall two percentiles below the mean on a standardized growth chart (2,3).

Treatment of failure to thrive depends on the cause, and begins with a careful assessment of medical status, growth patterns, and feeding issues (3). An interdisciplinary approach to evaluation and treatment is important. Feeding behavior, environmental conditions, and interaction with the parent or caregiver should be observed (4). The frequency and volume of feedings, occurrence of emesis after feedings, and the number of wet diapers and stools is important to ascertain. In formula fed infants, the diet history should include formula preparation method, since improper formula mixing can lead to both poor growth and fluid and electrolyte imbalances.

The ultimate goal in nourishing infants and children is to provide adequate energy for growth. In infants, this can be accomplished by concentrating the formula in increments up to 30 kcals/ounce. Breastmilk can be supplemented with milk fortifiers or powdered formula and given by bottle. Alternatively, either formula or breastmilk can be supplemented with modular calorie supplements providing primarily extra macronutrients, especially when renal solute load is an issue (3). The standard dilution for formulas is 20 kcals/ounce, which is generally prepared by mixing 1 scoop of powder with 2 ounces of water (4). Standard formulas mixed in this fashion provide 8–9% of the kcals as protein, so that 5 ounces of formula provides 100 kcals and

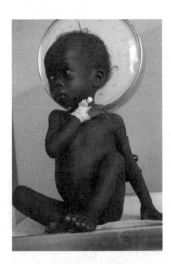

2.1–2.2 grams of protein. Manufacturers provide specific instructions for mixing both standard and more concentrated formulas.

The infant girl presented to a pediatric medical day program at age 8 months. She was born at 37 weeks gestation via vaginal delivery without complications at birth. Birth weight was 1989 grams. Diagnoses upon admission to the rehabilitation facility included a history of hydrocephalus with ventriculoperitoneal (VP) shunt at age 2 months, tetralogy of Fallot status post-repair at age 3 months, gastroesophageal reflux, and failure to thrive.

NUTRITIONAL ASSESSMENT DATA

1. Anthropometric Measurements.

Birth

Weight: 1989 g
Length: 49.2 cm
Head circumference: 34.8 cm

6 Months

Weight: (5.75 months of age): 4.9 kg
Length: (5.75 months of age): 65.5 cm
Head circumference: (5.75 months of age): 40.6 cm

At presentation to medical daycare (8 months)

Weight: 5.4 kg
Length: 66.04 cm
Head circumference: 41.6 cm

2. Biochemical Data.

Parameter	Value	Normal Range* (may vary by age, sex, and lab)
Sodium	139 mEq/L	139–146 mEq/L
Potassium	4.2 mEq/L	4.1–5.3 mEq/L
Chloride	98 mEq/L	98–106 mEq/L
Carbon dioxide	30 mEq/L	21–30 mEq/L
BUN	6 mg/dL	5–18 mg/dl
Creatinine	0.5 mg/dL	0.3–0.7 mg/dL

(continues)

(Continued)

Parameter	Value	Normal Range* (may vary by age, sex, and lab)
Glucose	81 mg/dL	50–90 mg/dL
Calcium	9.5 mg/dL	9.0–10.9 mg/dL
Phosphorus	6.0 mg/dL	4.3–9.3 mg/dL
Hemoglobin	11.8 g/dL	10.5–13.0 g/dL
Hematocrit	36.4%	33%–38%
Albumin	4.3 g/dL	4.0–5.0 g/dL

*Data from Herbold NH, Edelstein S. *Dietitian's Pocket Guide to Nutrition.* Sudbury, MA: Jones & Bartlett Learning; 2010: 401–414.

Data are from one week prior to first visit. Liver function tests and thyroid indices were reported as normal by the physician.

3. Nutrition-Focused Physical Findings.

She appears wasted. She has no edema or skin breakdown.

4. Client History.

Social History

The baby lives in an apartment with her parents, who are of Eastern European descent, and an 18-year-old brother. Mom speaks limited English; however, her older son is fluent in English. The mother is employed full-time and the baby's father is also employed, working the evening shift. Family history is unremarkable.

5. Food/Nutrition-Related History.

Reported Intake

Upon presentation the infant was drinking a standard milk-based formula with iron prescribed at a concentration of 24 kcal/oz. Mom reports she was mixing the formula by adding 2 scoops of formula to 4 ounces of water. Preadmission intake records also indicate patient drinking 1 ounce water daily and 1 ounce chamomile tea daily.

Three day nutritional intake records for formula volume were provided by the Mom upon admission:

Day 1 – 810 mL formula

Day 2 – 840 mL formula
Day 3 – 820 mL formula

Medications

Digoxin (0.05 mg/mL) 0.5 mL PO BID
Polyviflor (0.25 mg Fl per mL) 1 mL daily PO
Tylenol 10 mg/kg per dose PO every 4 hours PRN for pain or fever
> 101°F

QUESTIONS

1. Define low birthweight and very-low birthweight in grams. How would you classify this infant's birthweight? Was she premature or would she have been considered a full-term baby?
2. What growth chart(s) would you use to assess this infant's length and weight? Plot her growth on the chart from birth to 6 months and 8 months. What trends do you notice? What percentiles does she fall into for weight, length, and head circumference?
3. How would you determine her ideal body weight (IBW) based on her length, and what percentage of her IBW is she currently?
4. What is hydrocephalus and how might its presence affect anthropometric measurements, specifically head circumference? What is a ventriculoperitoneal (VP) shunt?
5. What is tetralogy of Fallot and how might it affect nutrition?
6. Explain the concept of "catch up growth" and how calorie and protein needs can be calculated when growth is less than optimal. What would you determine as calorie and protein needs for this child and why? Is she meeting her needs based on the volume of formula consumed and the mixing technique used (why or why not)?
7. What could you do to help her gain weight and grow properly? What questions would you ask regarding current feeding practices and tolerance? Would enteral feedings be appropriate for this baby (why or why not)?
8. What is the usual progression from breast or bottle to table foods? Is her intake appropriate for a normally developed infant of her age? Assuming that she has developmental delays, how would you approach oral feedings with this infant?

9. Identify an appropriate Nutrition Diagnosis and write a PES statement based on the available nutritional assessment data.
10. How would you monitor the effectiveness of your intervention?

REFERENCES AND SUGGESTED READINGS

1. Oomens PF. Severe failure to thrive in infancy: a case study. *Support Line.* 2004; 6:22–28.
2. Locklin M. The redefinition of failure to thrive from a case study perspective. *Pediatr Nursing.* 2005; 31:6, 474–495.
3. Rabinowitz SS, Bhatia J. *Nutritional Considerations in Failure to Thrive* (updated May 4, 2010). eMedicine from WebMD. Accessed April 18, 2011, from http://emedicine.medscape.com/article/985007-overview
4. Samour PQ, King K. *Pediatric Nutrition.* 4th ed. Sudbury, MA: Jones & Bartlett Learning, 2012.
5. Herbold NH, Edelstein S. *Dietitian's Pocket Guide to Nutrition.* Sudbury, MA: Jones & Bartlett Learning; 2010: 401–414.
6. Kleinman, RE, ed. Failure to thrive. In: *Pediatric Nutrition Handbook.* 6th ed. Elk Grove Village, IL: American Academy of Pediatrics; 2009: 601–636.
7. Center for Disease Control and Prevention (CDC). *WHO Growth Standards Are Recommended for Use in the U.S. for Infants and Children 0 to 2 Years of Age.* Accessed April 18, 2011, from http://www.cdc.gov/growthcharts/who_ charts.htm
8. Maqbool A, Olsen IE, and Stallings VA. Clinical Assessment of Nutritional Status. In: *Nutrition in Pediatrics,* 4th ed. Hamilton, Ontario, Canada: BC Decker Inc.; 2008: 5–14.
9. Kramer LC, Reinolds M. *Spina Bifida Hydrocephalus, and Shunts* (updated April 2011). eMedicine from WebMD. Accessed April 18, 2011, from http://emedicine.medscape.com/article/937979-overview
10. Spekor M, Dunson DA, Pflieger K. *Tetralogy of Fallot in Emergency Medicine* (updated December 2009). eMedicine from WebMD. Accessed April 18, 2011, from http://emedicine.medscape.com/article/760387-overview
11. Barness LA, Dallman PR, Anderson H, et al. On the feeding of supplemental foods to infants. *Pediatrics* 1980; 65:1178–1181.
12. Butte N, Cobb K, Dwyer J, Graney L, Heird W, Rickard K. The start healthy feeding guidelines for infants and toddlers. *J Am Diet Assoc.* 2004; 104:3, 442–454.
13. American Dietetic Association (ADA), *International Dietetics & Nutrition Terminology (IDNT) Reference Manual: Standardized Language for the Nutrition Care Process,* 3rd ed. Chicago, IL: ADA; 2010.

Food Allergies in a Toddler

LEARNING OBJECTIVES

Upon completing this case study, readers will be able to:

1. Describe food allergies and their nutritional management.
2. Plot and interpret pediatric anthropometric measures.
3. Assess the nutritional status of a patient with multiple food allergies.
4. Suggest appropriate dietary interventions for a patient with multiple food allergies.

CASE DESCRIPTION/BACKGROUND

Ensuring adequate growth of children is one of the foundations of pediatric dietetics. Absolute values of length or height, weight, and head circumference as well as BMI or weight-for-length plotted on appropriate growth charts are valuable indicators (1). It is also important to follow growth velocity trends.

Food allergy is defined as a reaction of the immune system after eating a certain food. Food allergies are classified into IgE-mediated, non-IgE mediated, and mixed IgE mediated diseases. In immunoglobulin E

(IgE)-mediated disease, the immune system is involved in the body's response to proteins. The major IgE-mediated allergic diseases are oral allergy syndrome, anaphylaxis, urticaria (hives), and angioedema; the most serious of which is anaphylaxis. Non-IgE mediated disease includes food protein-induced enterocolitis syndrome (FPIES), protein-induced enteropathy, and gluten-sensitive enteropathy (Celiac disease) (1). Although non-IgE mediated diseases are not technically allergies, food avoidance is necessary and therefore nutrition management is similar. Because there is currently no cure available for food allergy, strict avoidance of the offending protein is the only solution.

Allergy skin testing is commonly used to assess whether elimination of certain foods are indicated. In a child over one year old, a negative skin test is 95% predictive that a child is not allergic. However, only around 40% of children will experience allergic symptoms if they ingest a food for which they had a positive skin test (2). A food challenge in the allergist's office is the definitive way to determine whether a child will have an allergic reaction to a food.

Food allergies were reported in 3.9% of children in the United States in 2007, up 10% over the previous ten years (3). Children with two or

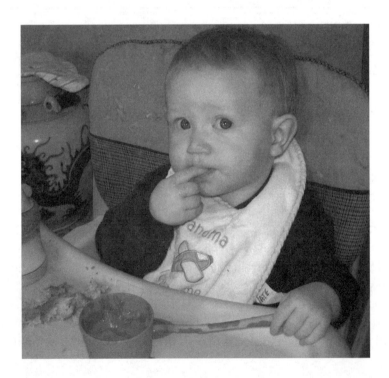

more food allergies were found to be shorter and at risk for inadequate intake for multiple nutrients than those with only one food allergy (4). Nutrient requirements for children with food allergies are not different than requirements for children without food allergies (4). In-depth nutrition education must be given to families for successful dietary elimination, including label reading, cross-contamination, restaurant dining, and nutrient replacement (4). For each allergenic food category, care must be taken to identify macronutrients and micronutrients provided by the food; appropriate food substitutes and supplements should be recommended (1).

The client is a 14-month-old boy who presented with weight maintenance and falling growth percentiles. The patient had been breastfed exclusively for the first five months of life when single-ingredient foods had been introduced twice per week with no reactions. The patient continued to be breastfed until one year. Egg white, cow milk protein, and peanuts had not been introduced before one year of age. Upon introduction of both cow's milk and eggs, the patient developed hives and eczema. The child visited an allergist who diagnosed milk, egg, and peanut allergy via skin test. Mom has eliminated these foods from the child's diet and has been giving rice milk because she read on the Internet that soy milk can cause boys to become feminized.

His mother states that he has been taking longer naps and has been more irritable lately. He is seeing the registered dietitian today because he has failed to gain weight and his weight-for-length measurement has crossed one percentile range.

NUTRITIONAL ASSESSMENT DATA

1. Anthropometric Measurements.

12-Month Visit

Length: 78 cm
Weight: 9 kg
Head circumference: 48 cm

Current Data (14 Months)

Length: 80 cm
Weight: 9 kg
Head circumference: 48.3 cm

2. Nutrition-Focused Physical Findings.

Vital signs: Blood pressure within normal limits.
The patient appears thin and lethargic. He has dark circles under
  his eyes.

3. Client History.

Social History

The patient lives with his parents, 7-year-old sister, and a dog. He is not a
picky eater.

4. Food/Nutrition-Related History.

The following represents his usual intake:

Meal	Time	Description
Breakfast	8 AM	½ cup oatmeal made with water, ¼ cup sliced strawberries, 4 oz original (unfortified) rice milk
Snack	10 AM	6 cut up grapes, 4 oz water
Lunch	Noon	2 tbs hummus with ½ pita bread, 4 oz unsweetened applesauce, 4 oz water
Snack	3 PM	4 rice wafers, 4 oz apple juice
Dinner	5:30 PM	½ cup angel hair pasta with ¼ cup tomato sauce, 4 oz original (unfortified) rice milk, ½ cup gelatin dessert
Snack	8 PM	½ cup diced canned peaches in juice, 8 oz water

Medications

None

Supplements

None

QUESTIONS

1. Define food allergy and describe common symptoms. List
   common food allergens.
2. What is the difference between a food allergy, such as milk
   protein allergy, and a food intolerance, such as lactose
   intolerance?

3. Plot this child's weight, length, weight-for-length, and head circumference on the CDC growth chart based on WHO growth standards (see Appendix C1 for link to charts).
4. How would you categorize this patient's growth pattern? What is his percentage of IBW at one year and 14 months? What are your concerns about his growth pattern?
5. List his requirements for kcals, protein, fat, calcium, Vitamin D, iron, and zinc.
6. How does his diet compare to the recommendations in question #5? Justify your answer by comparing his calorie, protein, fat, calcium, Vitamin D, iron, and zinc intake to recommended levels. Show your work.
7. Suggest specific modifications of diet that might improve this patient's health. What education should be given to the family?
8. Write a revised one-day meal plan based on his usual intake. Show nutrient levels to indicate that the new meal plan meets his needs for the nutrients in questions #5 and #6.
9. Write a PES statement that would apply to this patient.
10. What are your overall goals for this client, and how would you monitor the effectiveness of your interventions?

REFERENCES AND SUGGESTED READINGS

1. Corkins MR, Balint J, Bobo E, Plogsted S, Yaworski JA. *The A.S.P.E.N. Pediatric Nutrition Support Core Curriculum.* Silver Spring, MD: American Society of Parenteral and Enteral Nutrition; 2010.
2. Bock SA. Diagnostic evaluation. *Pediatrics.* 2003; 111:1638–1644.
3. Branum AM, Lukacs SL. Food allergy among children in the United States. *Pediatrics.* 2009; 124:1549–1555.
4. Mofidi S. Nutritional management of pediatric food hypersensitivity. *Pediatrics.* 2003; 111:1645–1653.
5. Christie L, Hine RJ, Parker JG, Burks W. Food allergies in children affect nutrient intakes and growth. *J Am Diet Assoc.* 102; 11:1648–1651.
6. Badger TM, Gilchrist JM, Pivik RT, Andres A, et al. The health implications of soy infant formula. *Am J Clin Nutr* 2009;89(Suppl); 1668S–1672S.
7. American Dietetic Association (ADA). *International Dietetics & Nutrition Terminology (IDNT) Reference Manual: Standardized Language for the Nutrition Care Process,* 3rd ed. Chicago, IL: ADA; 2010.

Childhood Obesity

LEARNING OBJECTIVES

Upon completing this case study, readers will be able to:

1. Describe risk factors associated with the development of obesity in children.
2. Identify factors affecting the development of obesity in an individual child.
3. Utilize nutrition assessment techniques to evaluate an overweight child.
4. Suggest appropriate interventions for weight management in children.

CASE DESCRIPTION/BACKGROUND

Obesity rates have increased in all pediatric age groups in the National Health and Nutrition Examination Surveys conducted in the United States since the 1970s (1). Between 1976–1980 and 2007–2008, the prevalence of obesity increased from 5.0% to 10.4% for ages 2 to 5 years, from 6.5% to 19.6% among those ages 6 to 11 years, and from 5.0% to

18.1% among adolescents ages 12 to 19 years (2). Obesity in children over 2 years is defined as a BMI greater than the 95th percentile for age when plotted on sex-specific Centers for Disease Control and Prevention (CDC) 2000 growth charts (3).

Childhood obesity is associated with metabolic dysfunction including impaired glucose tolerance, type 2 diabetes, and high cholesterol, triglyceride, and insulin levels (4). Children and adolescents who become obese are more likely to be obese as adults thereby having a higher lifetime risk of cardiovascular disease and cancer (5). The primary cause of obesity is energy intake greater than energy expenditure. Many secondary individual and environmental factors affect the primary cause of obesity, but it is unknown which specific ones put children, either individually or as a group, at the greatest risk for high energy intake and limited energy expenditure (6).

Genetic variation may predispose some children to obesity (7). In an individual child, neuroendocrine signals that control appetite or energy homeostasis have been shown to affect body weight (8). Individual factors also include what and how much food the child eats and whether they get regular exercise either through sports, play, or school (9). Dietary factors and eating behaviors that place children and adolescents at increased risk of obesity are consumption of calorically-sweetened beverages, lack of breakfast, increased frequency of eating out, low calcium intake, high total dietary fat intake, and increased portion size of meals. Increased fruit and vegetable intake is associated with decreased risk of child obesity (10,11). It is currently unknown whether snacking behavior in children is associated with obesity. However, children currently consume more than 27% of daily calories from snacks (12). Increased availability of high-calorie, nutrient-poor foods at home is associated with increased consumption of those types of snacks (13).

Parenting style and family environment is also associated with child obesity. Parental over-restriction of nutrient-poor foods and parental concern about the child's weight is associated with increased risk of obesity. Factors that create a negative family environment such as lack of parental time or support increase the risk of child obesity. In contrast, positive family environments where children have parental support and can appropriately express themselves decrease the risk (10,12). Increased time watching television and playing video games is associated with child obesity; television viewing is also associated with increased energy intake due to food advertisements. Increased physical activity and participation in sports is associated with decreased risk of obesity in children (10,11).

Community and social factors also affect the development of obesity in children. Whether a community has health-promoting food available for purchase and provides walkable areas affects obesity rates (14). Federal school wellness policies and programs aimed at increasing activity and decreasing high calorie food consumption at school have had some impact in decreasing child obesity in some areas of the United States but not enough to help overall obesity rates decline due to varying local resources (15).

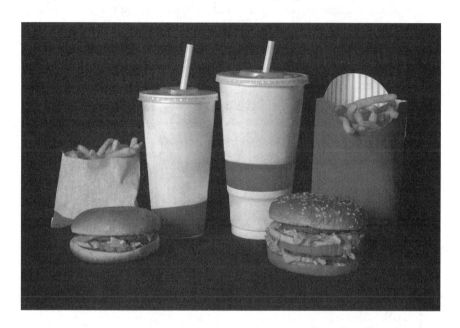

The patient is a 9½–year-old girl. She was referred for weight loss in your outpatient weight management program. She has been diagnosed with asthma and complains of shortness of breath while exercising, so tends to avoid it. She has no other medical history. The patient lives with her mother, baby sister, two brothers, and grandmother in a suburban neighborhood. The mother is single and works to support the family. The grandmother cooks for the family and takes care of the patient and her siblings after school until her mother gets home. Mom is also obese but grandmother and the siblings are normal weight.

The patient's school district has recently cut its physical education programs. The client enjoys playing outside after school, but her grandmother makes her come inside after a short time to do homework. After homework she is allowed to watch TV. The total time that she spends in front of the computer or TV is 4 to 6 hours per day. When not watching TV, she enjoys reading as a hobby.

Grandmother cooks approximately 4 nights per week and the family eats out or obtains take-out food for the remaining 3 nights. The client eats two helpings of food at dinner and will eat multiple helpings of snacks if left unattended. She drinks fruit drinks or similar calorie-containing beverages for thirst. Her favorite snacks are cookies and ice cream. She does not like vegetables but will eat fruit when available. Most snacks available in the house are purchased at a large discount store. Mom buys fruit from the local farmer's market once per week but the amount that is affordable only lasts a few days.

NUTRITIONAL ASSESSMENT DATA

1. Anthropometric Measurements.

Height: 4'9" (57")
Weight: 132 lbs

2. Biochemical Data.

Lab	Result	Normal Range* (may vary by age, sex, and lab)
Triglyceride	190 mg/dL	35–114 mg/dL
Total Cholesterol	160 mg/dL	120–200 mg/dL

*Data from Herbold NH, Edelstein S. *Dietitian's Pocket Guide to Nutrition*. Sudbury, MA: Jones & Bartlett Learning; 2010: 401–414.

3. Nutrition-Focused Physical Findings.

Vital signs: Blood pressure: 132/90 (normal 107/57) (16)
Heart rate: Normal

The patient is an active, alert child with significant excess body fatness. Her physical exam is overall normal except for reporting fatigue and shortness of breath with physical activity. Her thyroid function tests were within normal limits. The client's mother is noted to be obese.

4. Client History.

Social History

The patient is a shy child who prefers reading to social activities or team sports. She is a good student and participates in a local Girl Scout troop. She reports one best friend but otherwise has a limited friendship circle and reports being teased often about her weight.

5. Food/Nutrition-Related History.

Usual Diet

Meal	Description
Breakfast	1 bowl of cereal with 2% milk or 1 toaster pastry
	8 oz glass of orange juice
Snack	1 snack package of mini-muffins
	16 oz bottle of juice drink
Lunch	School lunch offering
	16 oz bottle of soda from vending machine
	Note: The patient reports that she does not like milk from school lunch because it tends to be warm and tastes bad.
	Cookie or ice cream (bought as extra to school lunch)
Snack	Snack chips or pretzels
	16 oz bottle of juice drink
	Grazes on various snacks available at home until dinner; sometimes includes fruit if available
Dinner	Chicken or beef – 4 oz
	Potatoes – 1 cup mashed or oven baked with oil
	Broccoli or peas – ½ cup
	Salad – 1 bowl with 2 tbs Thousand Island dressing
	2 pieces of bread with 1 tbs tub margarine
	8 oz 2% milk
	Note: Often has second helpings of meat and potatoes.
Snack	Snack cake, cookies, ice cream bar – whatever is in the house
	Note: Family purchases large packages of snack foods and juice drinks from a discount food club. Individual snack packages average 250 calories each and drinks come in 16 oz bottles.

Medications

Cromolyn sodium inhaler for asthma

Supplements

None

QUESTIONS

1. Plot the client's weight, height, and BMI on a CDC growth chart for girls, ages 2 to 20. Calculate and interpret her BMI.
2. The primary cause of obesity is energy imbalance. What factors within the patient's individual, family, or community environment may affect energy balance?
3. Describe the general principles of weight management in children in regard to energy intake.
4. Describe the general principles of weight management in children in regard to energy expenditure.
5. Write a PES statement for this case.
6. What specific recommendations would you make for this child and her family?
7. How would you monitor the outcome of your intervention?
8. What community resources would you suggest to this family to help them achieve and maintain normal body weight?
9. What factors may hinder compliance with healthy lifestyle recommendations in this family?
10. Please write a note summarizing your assessment in ADIME and SOAP format.

REFERENCES AND SUGGESTED READINGS

1. Bell J, Rogers VW, Dietz WH, Ogden CL, Schuler C, Popovic T. CDC Grand Rounds: childhood obesity in the United States. *Morbid Mortal Wkly Rep MMWR.* 2011; 60(2):42–46.
2. Ogden C, Carroll M. *Prevalence of Obesity Among Children and Adolescents: United States, Trends 1963-1965 Through 2007-2008.* CHS Health E-Stat, Centers for Disease Control and Prevention (CDC) (June 2010). Accessed April 18, 2011, from http://www.cdc.gov/nchs/data/hestat/obesity_child_07_08/obesity_child_07_08.htm

3. Division of Nutrition, Physical Activity, and Obesity, National Center for Chronic Disease Prevention and Health Promotion. *Defining Childhood Overweight and Obesity.* Center for Disease Control and Prevention (CDC) (2009). Accessed April 18, 2011, from http://www.cdc.gov/obesity/childhood/defining.html

4. St. Onge M-P, Keller KL, Heymsfield SB. Changes in childhood food consumption patterns: a cause for concern in light of increasing body weights. *Am J Clin Nutr.* 2003; 78:1068–1073.

5. Biro FM, Wien M. Childhood obesity and adult morbidities. *Am J Clin Nutr.* 2010; 91:1499S–1505S.

6. Trasande L, Cronk C, Durkin M, Weiss M, Schoeller D. Environment and obesity in the National Children's Study. *Environ Health Perspect.* 2009; 117:159–166.

7. Perusse L, Bouchard C. Gene-diet interactions in obesity. *Am J Clin Nutr.* 2000; 72:1285S–1290S.

8. Morrison C, Berthoud H. Neurobiology of nutrition and obesity. *Nutr Rev.* 2007; 65:517–553.

9. Ebbeling C, Pawlak D, Ludwig D. Childhood obesity: public health crisis, common sense cure. *Lancet.* 2002; 360:473–482.

10. American Dietetic Association (ADA). *American Dietetic Association Pediatric Weight Management Evidence-Based Nutrition Practice Guideline.* Chicago, IL: ADA; 2007.

11. Ritchie L, Welk G, Styne D, Gerstein D, Crawford P. Family environment and pediatric overweight: what is a parent to do? *J Am Diet Assoc.* 2005; 105:570–579.

12. Piernas C, Popkin B. Trends in snacking among U.S. children. *Health Aff.* 2010; 29:398–404.

13. Campbell K, Crawford D, Salmon J, Carver A, Garnett S, Baur L. Associations between home food environment and obese-promoting eating behaviors in adolescence. *Obesity.* 2007; 15(3):719–730.

14. Zick C, Smith K, Fan J, Brown B, Yamada I, Kowaleski-Jones L. Running to the store? The relationship between neighborhood environments and the risk of obesity. *Soc Sci Med.* 2009; 69(10):1493-1500.

15. Probart C, McDonnal ET, Jomaa L, Fekete V. Lessons from Pennsylvania's mixed response to federal school wellness law. *Health Aff.* 2010; 29:447–453.

16. Eckvall SW, Ekvall VK, eds. *Pediatric Nutrition in Chronic Diseases and Developmental Disorders: Prevention, Assessment, and Treatment,* 2nd ed. Oxford University Press; 2005:136–144.

17. American Dietetic Association (ADA). *International Dietetics & Nutrition Terminology (IDNT) Reference Manual: Standardized Language for the Nutrition Care Process,* 3rd ed. Chicago, IL: American Dietetic Association; 2010.

Cardiovascular Disease

Weight Management for Metabolic Syndrome

LEARNING OBJECTIVES

Upon completing this case study, readers will be able to:

1. Interpret anthropometric measurements of obesity.
2. Apply basic nutritional and dietary assessment skills.
3. Recognize signs of metabolic syndrome.
4. Discuss stages of health behavior change.
5. Suggest diet and exercise changes to assist in weight management and amelioration of symptoms of metabolic syndrome.

CASE DESCRIPTION AND BACKGROUND

Overweight and obesity are significant problems in the United States, with 68% of Americans over age 20 considered either overweight or obese, and half of those (34%) considered to be obese (1). These statistics are based on measurements of adult subjects using a definition of BMI ≥ 25 kg/m^2 for overweight and ≥ 30 kg/m^2 for obesity (1). Obesity rates vary among sex, age, and race, and there is some debate about the relative risk for obesity-related problems within various subsets of the population. Nonetheless, obesity is a known risk factor for metabolic syndrome and chronic diseases such as type 2 diabetes, hypertension, heart disease, stroke, some types of cancer, and arthritis (1,2).

Metabolic syndrome is a group of risk factors associated with obesity and insulin resistance that include: abdominal obesity, hyperlipidemia, high blood pressure, insulin resistance with or without glucose intolerance, prothrombic state, and proinflammatory state (3,4). Underlying causes of metabolic syndrome include overweight/obesity, physical inactivity, and a genetic predisposition (4). Metabolic syndrome increases the risk of coronary heart disease and type 2 diabetes. According to the National Cholesterol Education Panel's Adult Treatment Panel (ATP) III report (4), the diagnosis of metabolic syndrome is made when a patient displays at least three of the following five risk factors:

1. Waist circumference > 40 inches in men and 35 inches in women
2. Serum triglycerides ≥ 150 mg/dL
3. HDL cholesterol < 40 mg/dL in men and < 50 mg/dL in women
4. Blood pressure ≥ 130/≥ 85 mm Hg
5. Fasting glucose ≥ 110 mg/dL

Many factors contribute to obesity, overweight, and metabolic syndrome, including genetic, physiological, environmental, and behavioral

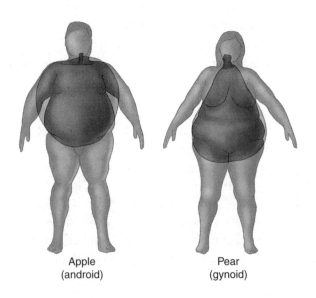

Apple
(android)

Pear
(gynoid)

factors. A combination of diet, physical activity, and behavioral therapy is generally recommended for weight management (3,5). Merely giving individuals directives to change is usually ineffective; guiding clients to identify and set their own goals can help to promote behavior change (3,6).

The client is a 41-year-old mother of two teenage children. She was an athlete in high school and never worried about her weight at that time. During her college years, she stopped playing sports and gained approximately 20 pounds. After graduation, she lost 15 pounds before her wedding. She gained approximately 40 to 50 pounds with each pregnancy; the first baby was born at 8 pounds, 13 ounces and the second weighed 9 pounds at birth. She never lost all of the weight after her children were born. She tried various diets but never stuck to any, and her weight has fluctuated while gradually creeping up over the years. She does not engage in regular physical activity. She comes to you because her doctor has referred her for weight loss. She states, "I want to set a good example for my children, but I am too busy to exercise. The kids won't eat anything but junk and I don't want to make separate dinners."

NUTRITIONAL ASSESSMENT DATA

1. Anthropometric Measurements.

Height: 5'6"
Weight: 178 lbs
Weight at age 21: 140 lbs
Waist circumference: 38 inches

2. Biochemical Data.

The following results are fasting measures.

Parameter	Result	Reference Range* (may vary by age, sex, and lab)
Sodium	141 mEq/L	135–147 mEq/L
Potassium	4.8 mEq/L	3.5–5.0 mEq/L
Chloride	106 mEq/L	98–106 mEq/L
CO_2	22 mEq/L	21–30 mEq/L
BUN	13 mg/dL	8–23 mg/dL

(continues)

(Continued)

Parameter	Result	Reference Range* (may vary by age, sex, and lab)
Creatinine	0.7 mg/dL	0.7–1.5 mg/dL
Glucose (fasting)	126 mg/dL	70–110 mg/dL
Albumin	4.0 g/dL	3.5–5.5 g/dL
Hemoglobin	13.8 g/dL	14–18 g/dL (male) 12–16 g/dL (female)
Hematocrit	42%	38%–54% (male) 36%–47% (female)
Hemoglobin A1C	5.1%	4.0%–6.0%
Total cholesterol	193 mg/dL	< 200 mg/dL
HDL cholesterol	38 mg/dL	< 40 mg/dL (male) > 50 mg/dL (female)
LDL cholesterol	119 mg/dL	< 100 mg/dL with heart disease or diabetes < 130 mg/dL with risk factors
Triglyceride	189 mg/dL	< 150 mg/dL

*Data from U. S. Food and Drug Administration (FDA). *Investigations Operations Manual.* Silver Spring, MD: FDA; 2001. Accessed April 18, 2011, from http://www.fda.gov/downloads/ICECI/Inspections/IOM/UCM135835.pdf
Morris JC. *Dietitian's Guide to Assessment and Documentation.* Sudbury, MA: Jones & Bartlett Learning; 2011.

3. Nutrition-Focused Physical Findings.

The client is a well-developed, well-nourished woman. Blood pressure is 140/90 mm Hg. She complains of low energy levels.

4. Client History.

The client's grandmother and father were also obese. She does not smoke, and drinks occasionally.

5. Food/Nutrition-Related History.

Usual Diet

Breakfast

Skips; buys a latte or cappuccino after she drops the kids off at school.

Mid Morning Snack

Donut and 2% milk.

Lunch

Peanut butter and jelly sandwich on white bread with a piece of fruit. Drinks cola.

Afternoon Snack

Usually cookies and milk with the kids when they come home.

Dinner

Hamburgers or chicken, potato salad or scalloped potatoes, corn or peas. Green salad with ranch dressing. Ice cream or pudding or Jello for dessert. Drinks water.

Evening Snacks

Chips and dip, drinks juice.
She is not taking any medications. She takes a one-a-day multivitamin and no other supplements.

QUESTIONS

1. Describe the stages of readiness for change, and identify where you think she falls on this continuum.
2. Calculate her BMI. How would you interpret it? How does her waist circumference measurement add to your assessment?
3. What does her history of giving birth to heavier than average babies suggest?
4. Does she meet the criteria for this syndrome according to the National Cholesterol Education Panel's Adult Treatment Panel III? How is metabolic syndrome treated with diet and physical activity?
5. What can you do to help her become motivated from within herself to change her diet and exercise behaviors?
6. Assuming she becomes ready to take action, identify some initial steps that she might take to improve her diet.
7. What is the role of physical activity in weight loss and weight maintenance? How do aerobic activity, strength training, and stretching all contribute to optimal weight management?

8. What methods would you suggest she could use for self-monitoring?
9. Make suggestions for handling family meals, special occasions, and holidays.
10. Write a PES statement based on her initial presentation. How would you monitor and evaluate the effect of your interventions?

REFERENCES AND SUGGESTED READINGS

1. Flegal KM, Carroll MD, Ogden CL, et al. Prevalence and trends in obesity among U.S. adults, 1999–2008. *JAMA*. 2010; 303(3):235–241.
2. Malnick SDH, Knobler H. The medical complications of obesity *QJM*. 2006; 99(9):565–579.
3. Artinian NT, Fletcher GJ, Mozaffarian D, Kris-Etherton P, et al. Interventions to promote physical activity and dietary lifestyle changes for cardiovascular risk factor reduction in adults: a scientific statement from the American Heart Association. *Circulation*. 2010; 122:406–441.
4. American Heart Association (AHA). Third Report of the National Cholesterol Education Program (NCEP) Expert Panel on Detection, Evaluation, and Treatment of High Blood Cholesterol in Adults. *Circulation*. 2002; 106: 3143–3421.
5. Eckel RH. Nonsurgical management of obesity in adults. *N Engl J Med*. 2008; 358:1941–1950.
6. Rollnick S, Butler CC, Kinnersley P, Gregor J, Mash B. Motivational interviewing. *BMJ*. 2010; 340:1242–1246.
7. Grundy SM, Cleeman JI, Daniels SR, et al. Diagnosis and management of the metabolic syndrome: an American Heart Association/National Heart, Lung, and Blood Institute Scientific Statement. *Circulation*. 2005; 112:2735–2752.
8. Rollnick S, Mason P, Butler C. *Health Behavior Change, A Guide for Practitioners*. Philadelphia, PA: Churchill Livingtone; 1999.
9. Grundy SM, Brewer HB, Cleeman JI, Smith SC, Lenfant C. Definition of the metabolic syndrome. *Circulation*. 2004; 109:433–438.
10. Greene GW, Rossi SR, Rossi JS, Velicer WF, Fava JL, Prochaska JO. Dietary applications of the stages of change model. *J Am Diet Assoc*. 1999; 6:673–678.
11. Hillier TA, Pedula KL, Vesco KK. Excess gestational weight gain: modifying fetal macrosomia risk associated with maternal glucose. *Obstet Gynecol*. 2008; 112:1007–1014.
12. American Dietetic Association (ADA). *International Dietetics & Nutrition Terminology (IDNT) Reference Manual: Standardized Language for the Nutrition Care Process*, 3rd ed. Chicago, IL: American Dietetic Association; 2010.

Hypertension in a Middle-Aged Man

LEARNING OBJECTIVES

Upon completing this case study, readers will be able to:

1. Describe hypertension and its associated risks.
2. Assess the nutritional status of a patient with hypertension.
3. Explain the relationship between diet and hypertension.
4. Suggest appropriate dietary interventions for a patient with hypertension.
5. Identify goals of therapy and outcomes for monitoring and evaluation of a patient with hypertension.

CASE DESCRIPTION/BACKGROUND

Hypertension is the most common treatable risk factor for cardiovascular disease, stroke, and kidney disease. *Hypertension* is broadly defined as a blood pressure greater than 140 millimeters of mercury (mm Hg) systolic and 90 mm Hg diastolic blood pressure. It can be further classified as prehypertension, stage 1 hypertension, or stage 2 hypertension, depending on repeated systolic and diastolic readings (1). Lowering systolic blood

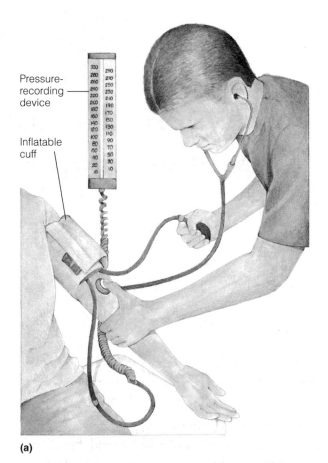

Pressure-recording device

Inflatable cuff

(a)

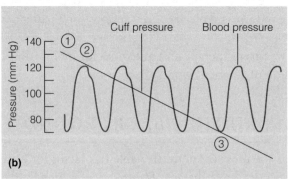

(b)

pressure by as little as 12 mm Hg over ten years in persons with hypertension and additional risk factors or disease is expected to prevent at least 1 death in every 9 to 11 persons treated (1). Weight control, physical activity, and the Dietary Approaches to Stop Hypertension (DASH) dietary pattern are helpful lifestyle modifications for controlling hypertension (2–4).

The client is a 60-year-old man with a type A personality. His colleagues consider him a workaholic. He arises at between 4:30 and 5:00 AM and works until 10 to 11 PM. His only relaxation is cooking, especially savory dishes with excessive salt. He exercises moderately by walking on a treadmill for approximately 20 minutes per day two to three times weekly. He comes to the registered dietitian for suggestions on ways to lower his blood pressure without taking additional antihypertensive medications.

NUTRITIONAL ASSESSMENT DATA

1. Anthropometric Measurements.

Height: 5′9″
Weight: 234 lbs

2. Biochemical Data.

Parameter	Value	Normal Range (*) (may vary by age, sex, and lab)
Sodium	136 mEq/L	135–147 mEq/L
Potassium	4.6 mEq/L	3.5–5.0 mEq/L
Chloride	103 mEq/L	98–106 mEq/L
Carbon dioxide	25 mEq/L	21–30 mEq/L
BUN	21 mg/dL	8–23 mg/dL
Creatinine	1.2mg/dL	0.7–1.5 mg/dL
Glucose	110 mg/dL	70–110 mg/dL
Albumin	4.2 g/dL	3.5–5.5 g/dL
Total cholesterol	238 mg/dL	< 200 mg/dL
LDL cholesterol	174 mg/dL	< 100 mg/dL with preexisting heart disease or diabetes < 130 mg/dL with heart disease risk factors

(continues)

(Continued)

Parameter	Value	Normal Range (*) (may vary by age, sex, and lab)	
HDL cholesterol	37 mg/dL	> 40 mg/dL men	*L*
		> 50 mg/dL women	
Triglycerides	133 mg/dL	< 150 mg/dL	

*Data from U. S. Food and Drug Administration (FDA). *Investigations Operations Manual.* Silver Spring, MD: U.S. FDA; 2001. Accessed April 19, 2011, from http://www.fda.gov/downloads/ICECI/Inspections/IOM/UCM135835.pdf

Morris JC. *Dietitian's Guide to Assessment and Documentation.* Sudbury, MA: Jones & Bartlett Learning; 2011.

American Heart Association. Third Report of the National Cholesterol Education Program (NCEP) Expert Panel on Detection, Evaluation, and Treatment of High Blood Cholesterol in Adults (Adult Treatment Panel III) Final Report. *Circulation.* 2002; 106:3143.

3. Nutrition-Focused Physical Findings.

Vital Signs

Blood pressure: 145/92
Heart rate: 71 bpm
Respirations: 18 rf

The patient is a balding gentleman who appears well nourished and on the heavy side. The remainder of the physical exam is normal except for some pain in his legs and feet, which limits his physical activity. *neuropathy*

4. Client History.

Social Hx

He does not smoke. He drinks alcohol socially.

5. Food/Nutrition-Related History.

Usual Diet

Meal	Description
Breakfast	Two large cups of coffee, each with 1 oz half and half,
	2 egg omelet with 1 oz American cheese; cooked in butter
	1 slice white toast with 1 tbs jelly

(Continued)

Meal	Description
Lunch	Deli sandwich, generally 4 oz ham and 2 oz Swiss cheese with 1 tbs mustard
Snack	Coffee with 1 oz half and half
Dinner	Grilled steak, approximately 8 oz seasoned generously with Montreal seasoning
	1 cup French fries with salt and 2 tbs catsup
	Iceberg lettuce with 2 slices crumbled bacon, 2 tbs blue cheese dressing
	16 oz diet tonic water
Snack	Ice cream, 1 cup premium

Medications

hydrochlorothiazide

Supplements

None

QUESTIONS

1. Define hypertension, suggest how his high blood pressure would be classified, and discuss how his hypertension affects his risk for future health problems.
2. What is his IBW, %IBW, and BMI? Estimate his caloric requirements. Show your work.
3. Explain the DASH diet. What levels of saturated fat, cholesterol, fiber, sodium, potassium, calcium, and magnesium are included? What would be an expected change in his blood pressure and blood lipids if he follows the DASH diet?
4. Analyze his diet using MyPyramid Tracker. How many kcals is he currently consuming, and how does this compare to his energy needs? How does his usual diet compare to the DASH recommendations?
5. What type of medication is he on for his blood pressure? Does it have any food–drug interactions?
6. Go to http://www.kidney.org/professionals/kdoqi/gfr_calculator .cfm and enter his age, race, gender, and creatinine level (check yes for "traceable to IDMS"). This calculates an estimated

glomerular filtration rate (GFR), which is a measure of kidney function. What is his estimated GFR (MDRD GFR in mL/min/1.73 m²)? If these readings persisted for at least three months, what would it suggest about the effects of hypertension on his kidneys?

7. Identify an appropriate nutrition diagnosis and write a PES statement.

8. Suggest specific modifications of diet and lifestyle (interventions) that might lower this client's blood pressure.

9. What are your overall goals for this client, and how would you monitor the results or outcomes of your interventions?

10. Write a note in ADIME or SOAP format that summarizes your assessment.

REFERENCES AND SUGGESTED READINGS

1. Chobanian AV, Bakris GL, Black HR, et al. Seventh report of the Joint National Committee on Prevention, Detection, Evaluation, and Treatment of High Blood Pressure. *Hypertension*. 2003; 42:1206–1252.

2. Sacks F, Campos H. Dietary therapy in hypertension. *N Engl J Med*. 2010; 362:2102–2112.

3. Lictenstein A, Appel L, Brands M, et al. Diet and lifestyle recommendations revision 2006. A scientific statement from the American Heart Association Nutrition Committee. *Circulation*. 2006; 114: 82–96.

4. Hill A, Fleming J, Kris-Etherton P. The role of diet and nutritional supplements in preventing and treating cardiovascular disease. *Curr Opin Cardiol*. 2009; 24:433–441.

5. Mifflin MD, St Jeor ST, Hill LA, Scott BJ, Daugherty SA, Koh YO. A new predictive equation for resting energy expenditure in healthy individuals. *Am J Clin Nutr*. 1990; 51(2):241–247.

6. MyPyramid Tracker. Alexandria, VA: USDA Center for Nutrition Policy and Promotion; 2009. Accessed April 19, 2011, from http://www.mypyramidtracker.gov

7. U.S. Department of Health and Human Services (DHHS), National Institutes of Health (NIH), and National Heart, Lung, and Blood Institute (NHLBI). *Your Guide to Lowering Your Blood Pressure With DASH*. NIH Publication No. 06-4082. Bethesda, MD: National Institutes of Health (revised 2006). Accessed April 19, 2011, from http://www.nhlbi.nih.gov/health/public/heart/hbp/dash/new_dash.pdf

8. Medline Plus. *Hydrochlorothiazide.* Bethesda, MD: National Library of Medicine (NLM); November 18, 2010. Accessed April 19, 2011, from http://www.nlm.nih.gov/medlineplus/druginfo/meds/a682571.html

9. National Kidney Foundation. *Frequently Asked Questions about GFR Estimates.* New York, NY: National Kidney Foundation; 2010. Accessed April 19, 2011, from http://www.kidney.org/professionals/kls/pdf/KBA_FAQs_AboutGFR .pdf

10. American Dietetic Association (ADA). *International Dietetics & Nutrition Terminology (IDNT) Reference Manual: Standardized Language for the Nutrition Care Process*, 3rd ed. Chicago, IL: ADA; 2010.

Heart Failure in an Obese Woman

LEARNING OBJECTIVES

Upon completing this case study, readers will be able to:

1. Identify the role of nutrition therapy in the management of heart failure.
2. Interpret alterations in anthropometric and biochemical data during heart failure.
3. Apply basic nutritional and dietary assessment skills.
4. Utilize the Nutrition Care Process in a patient with heart failure and concurrent comorbid conditions.

CASE DESCRIPTION/BACKGROUND

Heart failure affects 4.9 million people in the United States, accounting for 12 to 15 million doctor's office visits and 6.5 million hospital admissions each year (1,2). It is one of the most common causes of hospitalization in the Medicare population, and is expected to grow in incidence as the elderly population expands (1,2). Although *heart failure* is the preferred term (2), the condition historically has been called *congestive heart failure (CHF)* and is commonly referred to as such. In heart failure, the heart's ability to pump blood is impaired, resulting in reduced cardiac output and poor perfusion of body tissues. Increased heart rate and vasoconstriction follow as the sympathetic nervous system becomes activated. The renin-angiotensin-aldosterone system is triggered, resulting in increased sodium and fluid retention as the body tries to compensate for reduced blood flow (3). This ultimately can lead to a worsening in cardiac function.

The four stages of heart failure are: Stages A and B, defined as asymptomatic patients with or without structural heart damage, respectively; Stage C, both structural and symptomatic heart failure; and Stage D, refractory heart failure (2). Because hospital readmissions are frequently related to noncompliance with treatments including diet (4) and because poor diet quality is common in this population (5), the registered dietitian should focus on sodium intake and fluid status in addition to adequate energy, protein, and micronutrient intake.

The patient is a 60-year-old woman with history of type 2 diabetes, Stage C heart failure, and temporal arteritis, for which she was recently started on oral steroids. She lives with her sister, who is responsible for cooking and food shopping. The sister also cared for their mother who had diabetes and has since passed away. The patient has limited mobility because of her heart failure and osteoarthritis, and does not work. She requires assistance with activities of daily living. She is admitted to the hospital with a chief complaint of shortness of breath, orthopnea, fatigue, and swelling of her legs. She is diagnosed with exacerbation of heart failure

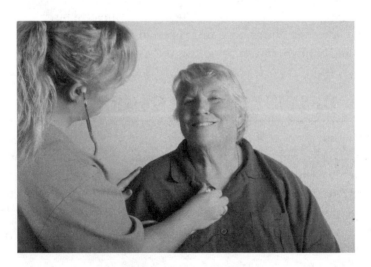

based on her symptoms and an elevated BNP (B-type or brain natriuretic peptide). BNP is a hormone that is released by the heart into the blood when the left ventricle is stretched and cardiac output falls. BNP can be used to differentiate between pulmonary and cardiac causes of dyspnea (5–7). The physician prescribes an 1800 kilocalorie, 2 gram sodium, low-fat diet, and consults the registered dietitian.

NUTRITIONAL ASSESSMENT DATA

1. Anthropometric Measurements.

Height: 5'7"
Weight: 245.5 lbs
Usual weight: 230 lbs. Gained approximately 15 lbs in 2 weeks prior to admission.

2. Biochemical Data, Medical Tests, and Procedures.

a. Labs

Parameter	Value	Normal Range* (may vary by age, sex, and lab)	
Sodium	137 mEq/L	135–147 mEq/L	
Potassium	4.8 mEq/L	3.5–5.0 mEq/L	
Chloride	103 mEq/L	98–106 mEq/L	
Carbon dioxide	31 mEq/L	21–30 mEq/L	H
BUN	25 mg/dL	8–23 mg/dL	H
Creatinine	1.2 mg/dL	0.7–1.5 mg/dL	
Glucose	237 mg/dL	70–110 mg/dL	H
Hemoglobin	11.3 g/dL	12–16 g/dL (woman)	L
Hematocrit	36%	36–47% (woman)	
Albumin	3.0 g/dL	3.5–5.5 g/dL	L
Magnesium	1.9 mEq/L	1.8–3.6 mEq/L	
Phosphorus	3.5 mg/dL	3.0–4.5 mg/dL	
BNP	450 pg/mL	< 100 pg/mL	H

*Data from U. S. Food and Drug Administration (FDA). *Investigations Operations Manual.* Silver Spring, MD: U.S. FDA; 2001. Accessed April 19, 2011, from http://www.fda.gov/downloads/ICECI/Inspections/IOM/UCM135835.pdf
Morris JC. *Dietitian's Guide to Assessment and Documentation.* Sudbury, MA: Jones & Bartlett Learning; 2011.

b. Test results, if pertinent

Point of care blood glucoses range from 213 to 291 mg/dL

3. Nutrition-Related Physical Findings.

She appears obese, in no acute distress. Her skin is intact. She has bilateral lower extremity pitting edema to the knee. She is missing a few teeth but denies problems chewing or swallowing.

4. Client History.

Social Hx

No smoking or alcohol

Family Hx

The client reports that she has been diabetic since she was 40 years old. Her mother also had diabetes.

5. Food/Nutrition-Related History.

She states that her sister prepares breakfast and fixes a lunch for her before leaving for work, then prepares dinner when she returns from work. Patient reports that she does not use any sugar or salt.

Usual Diet

Breakfast

Cereal, corn flakes, 1½ cups
2% milk, 1 cup
Banana
Orange juice, 8 oz
Tea with artificial sweetener, 12-oz mug

Lunch

2 slices ham or bologna with 1 slice American cheese sandwich on
white bread with 1 tsp mustard
Diet Jello, ½ cup
Diet cola, one 12-oz can

Dinner

1 chicken patty, baked or broiled
½ cup mashed or baked potato with 1 tbs margarine
½ cup broccoli with 2 tbs ready-to-serve cheese sauce
Lettuce & tomato salad with 2 tbs bottled Italian dressing
Water, one 16-oz bottle
Pound cake, 1 slice with vanilla ice cream, 1 scoop

Snacks

She denies snacking through the day; she drinks an additional 12 to 16-oz of diet soda or water. Currently in the hospital, meal intake is recorded at 80% to100% consistently. She confirms that her appetite is good.

Medications

Aldactone 100 mg/day, Humulin 70/30, 70 units BID plus sliding
    scale insulin, prednisone 40 mg/day, lasix 40 mg/day

Supplements

None

QUESTIONS

1. Which weight would be most appropriate to use as a starting point in your nutritional assessment, the admission weight or her usual weight? Why?
2. Calculate and interpret her BMI. How would you determine the energy and protein needs of a HF patient? Estimate her needs, and show your work.
3. Do you think she would benefit from a multivitamin or any specific vitamin/mineral supplements? Why or why not?
4. What non-nutritional factors could be aggravating her hyperglycemia?
5. Why do you think her albumin is low in the face of a good appetite?
6. Estimate the sodium and fluid content of her usual diet using a nutrient database such as the one on the USDA website. Show your work.

7. How does her sodium and fluid intake compare with common sodium and fluid recommendations for diet in heart failure? What advice would you give her to improve her diet habits and help avoid exacerbations of congestive heart failure?
8. Would your recommendations on sodium and/or fluid change at all if this patient's appetite had been poor? Why or why not?
9. Write a PES statement based on the available nutritional assessment data.
10. Name a specific intervention(s) that would address her nutrition diagnosis, and specify how you would monitor its effectiveness. In addition to diet and fluid status, what other parameter might you monitor in a HF patient?

REFERENCES AND SUGGESTED READINGS

1. Jacobsen D, Sevin C. Improved care for patients with congestive heart failure. *Jt Comm J Qual Patient Saf*. 2008; 34(1):13–19.
2. Jessup M, Abraham WT, Casey DE, et al., for the 2005 Guideline Update for the Diagnosis and Management of Chronic Heart Failure in the Adult Writing Committee. 2009 Focused update: ACCF/AHA guidelines for the diagnosis and management of heart failure in adults: a report of the American College of Cardiology Foundation/American Heart Association Task Force on Practice Guidelines. *Circulation*. 2009; 119: 1977–2016.
3. Jackson G, Gibbs CR, Davies MK, Lip GYH. ABC of Heart Failure. *BMJ*. 2000; 320:167–170.
4. Kuehneman T, Saulsbury D, Splett P, Chapman D. Demonstrating the impact of nutrition intervention in a heart failure program. *J Am Diet Assoc*. 2002; 102:1790–1794.
5. Lemon SC, Olendzki B, Magner R, et al. The dietary quality of persons with heart failure in NHANES 1999–2006. *J Gen Intern Med*. 2009; 25(2): 135–140.
6. McCullough PA, Nowak RM, McCord J, et al. B-type natriuretic peptide and clinical judgment in emergency diagnosis of heart failure: analysis from Breathing Not Properly (BNP) Multinational Study. *Circulation*. 2002; 106:416–422.
7. Hobbs RE. Using BNP to diagnose, manage, and treat heart failure. *Cleve Clin J Med*. 2003; 70(4):333–336. Accessed April 19, 2011, from http://www.ccjm.org/content/70/4/333.full.pdf
8. Mueller C, Scholer A, Laule-Kiliam M, et al. Use of B-type natriuretic peptide in the evaluation and management of acute dyspnea. *N Engl J Med*. 2004; 350:7, 647–654.

9. American Dietetic Association Evidence Analysis Library. *ADA Heart Failure Evidence-Based Nutrition Practice Guideline.* Accessed April 19, 2011, from http://www.adaevidencelibrary.com/topic.cfm?cat=3249&alt_header=1&library=EBG

10. American Dietetic Association Evidence Analysis Library. In obese adults, what is the prediction accuracy and maximum overestimation and underestimation errors compared to measured resting metabolic rate when using the Mifflin-St. Jeor formula? Accessed April 19, 2011, from http://www.adaevidencelibrary.com/conclusion.cfm?conclusion_statement_id=244

11. Hanninen SA, Darling PB, Sole MJ, Barr A, Keith ME. The prevalence of thiamin deficiency in hospitalized patients with congestive heart failure. *J Am Coll Cardiol.* 2006: 47:354–361.

12. Fuhrman PM, Charney P, Mueller C. Hepatic proteins and nutrition assessment. *J Am Diet Assoc.* 2004; 104:1258-1264.

13. U.S. Department of Agriculture (USDA), Agricultural Research Service. USDA National Nutrient Database for Standard Reference, Release 23. *Nutrient Data Laboratory Home Page* (modified December 2010). Accessed April 19, 2011, from http://www.ars.usda.gov/nutrientdata

14. American Dietetic Association (ADA). *International Dietetics & Nutrition Terminology (IDNT) Reference Manual: Standardized Language for the Nutrition Care Process*, 3rd ed. Chicago: ADA; 2010.

Post-Stroke Nutrition Management

LEARNING OBJECTIVES

Upon completing this case study, readers will be able to:

1. Define common post-stroke alterations in nutrition.
2. Suggest an appropriate enteral feeding regimen for a post-stroke patient.
3. Describe normal phases of swallowing.
4. Identify common diets used in patients with dysphagia.
5. Transition a patient from enteral to oral feedings.

CASE DESCRIPTION/BACKGROUND

Stroke is the third leading cause of death in this country. There are 795,000 strokes per year, the majority occurring in patients over the age of 65 (1). Stroke occurs when blood flow to the brain is interrupted by a blood clot or ruptured blood vessel. Brain damage occurs as a result, compromising functions controlled by the area of the brain affected. Common impairments involve motor functions, speech, swallowing, communication, memory, emotion, and judgment. After a stroke, many patients will gradually improve and regain at least some of their previous function.

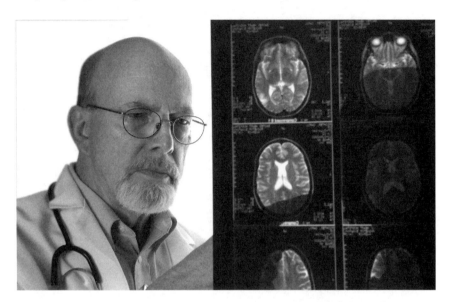

Risk factors for stroke are known and are generally divided into modifiable and non-modifiable risk factors. The non-modifiable risk factors are age, sex, and race. Modifiable risk factors include hypertension, smoking, diabetes, and hyperlipidemia. Because many of these modifiable risk factors are nutrition-related, diet can play an important role in the prevention of stroke (1).

Observational studies demonstrate that approximately 50% of stroke patients are undernourished on admission to the hospital (2,3) and therefore present with a compromised nutritional status. As many as 40% to 69% of stroke patients have dysphagia (4) and will require a feeding tube and/or dysphagia diet. For these patients, attention to nutrition is an important part of their acute recovery and long-term rehabilitation (5–7).

The client is a 77-year-old man who awoke from his sleep unable to move his right side or speak. He was brought to the emergency room where a computed tomography (CT) scan of the brain revealed a large left hemispheric stroke. He had a history of smoking, hypercholesterolemia, and hypertension. Because he awoke from sleep with his neurologic deficit, the time of onset of his stroke was not known. He was admitted to the hospital with the diagnosis of an acute left hemispheric stroke.

In the intensive care unit, he was evaluated for his ability to swallow by a speech-language pathologist. He was found to have delayed swallowing and pooling of oral secretions, and was therefore judged to be unsafe for an oral diet. A small bore nasogastric tube was placed for feeding given his dysphagia. During this time, the patient experienced increasing agitation and difficulty managing his oral secretions. He was intubated for airway protection and sedated with propofol. A consult from a registered dietitian was requested for recommendation of tube feedings.

Sedation was lifted and the patient was extubated after five days. He was moved from intensive care to a step-down unit. The tube feedings were continued, and he was re-evaluated by the speech pathologist. At this point the patient was controlling his oral secretions and exhibited minimal delay in swallowing. After a bedside swallowing evaluation, he was started on a pureed diet with pudding thick liquids.

NUTRITIONAL ASSESSMENT DATA

1. Anthropometric Measurements.

Height: 5'9"
Weight: 175 lbs (79 kg)

2. Biochemical Data and Test Results.

Laboratory results

Parameter	Value	Normal Range* (may vary by age, sex, and lab)
Sodium	141 mEq/L	135–147 mEq/L
Potassium	4.1 mEq/L	3.5–5.0 mEq/L
Chloride	110 mEq/L	98–106 mEq/L
Carbon dioxide	30 mEq/L	23–30 mEq/L
BUN	20 mg/dL	8–23 mg/dL
Creatinine	1.0 mg/dL	0.7–1.5 mg/dL
Glucose	100 mg/dL	70–110 mg/dL
Total cholesterol	216 mg/dL	< 200 mg/dL
LDL cholesterol	123 mg/dL	< 100 mg/dL with preexisting heart disease or diabetes < 130 mg/dL with heart disease risk factors

(continues)

(Continued)

Parameter	Value	Normal Range* (may vary by age, sex, and lab)
HDL cholesterol	30 mg/dL	> 40 mg/dL (men)
		> 50 mg/dL (women)
Triglycerides	173 mg/dL	< 150 mg/dL

*Data from: U. S. Food and Drug Administration (FDA). *Investigations Operations Manual*. Silver Spring, MD: US FDA; 2001. Accessed April 19, 2011, from http://www.fda.gov/downloads/ICECI/Inspections/IOM/UCM135835.pdf

Morris JC. *Dietitian's Guide to Assessment and Documentation*. Sudbury, MA: Jones & Bartlett Learning; 2011.

American Heart Association. Third report of the National Cholesterol Education Program (NCEP) Expert Panel on Detection, Evaluation, and Treatment of High Blood Cholesterol in Adults (Adult Treatment Panel III) Final Report. *Circulation* 2002; 106:3143.

3. Nutrition-Focused Physical Findings.

The patient is lethargic with global aphasia and right hemiparesis.

Vital Signs

Blood pressure: 180/95
Heart rate: 90 bpm
Temperature: 98.6°F

4. Client History.

Social Hx

Smokes ½ pack of cigarettes per day. Drinks alcohol socially. Patient is retired and lives alone.

5. Food/Nutrition-Related History.

Usual Diet

Unavailable on initial evaluation

Current Diet

NPO

Medications

The client was taking lisinopril, hydrochlorothiazide, and simvistatin at home. Upon initial evaluation, he was on normal saline at 60 mL/h and propofol at 15 mL/h. Diet was NPO.

Supplements

None

QUESTIONS

1. Define the terms dysphagia, aphasia, and hemiparesis.
2. What risk factors for stroke did the client have prior to admission?
3. Estimate his needs for calories, protein, and fluid.
4. How does the use of propofol affect your nutrition recommendations? What biochemical parameters should be checked when a patient is receiving propofol?
5. Suggest an enteral formula that would meet his needs. Assume that the IV fluids (saline) will be weaned by the physician as the enteral feeding advances. Specify how you would start the feeding and what the goal rate would be. At goal, how many calories and grams of protein are provided?
6. When sedation is lifted and the patient is extubated, what steps would you take to transition from enteral to oral feedings? How might the stroke itself, as well as the continuous enteral feedings, affect his ability to eat? What methods would you use to assess the adequacy of his oral food and beverage intake?
7. Describe the phases of normal swallowing.
8. Identify typical solid and liquid consistencies on the National Dysphagia Diet. Give examples of types of foods recommended on each diet.
9. Write a PES statement for him when he starts on the oral diet.
10. What are your goals for him once he is on the dysphagia diet, and how would you monitor and evaluate the outcome of your interventions?

REFERENCES AND SUGGESTED READINGS

1. Heart Disease and Stroke Statistics 2010 Update: A Report from the American Heart Association. *Circulation.* 2010; 121: e46–e215.
2. Bath PMW, Bath FJ, Smithard DG. Interventions for dysphagia in acute stroke. In: *The Cochrane Library.* Issue 3, 2004. Chichester, UK: John Wiley and Sons LTD.
3. Ray S, Rana P, Rajput M, Haleem M. Nutritional management of stroke: from current evidence to conjecture. *Nutr Bull.* 2007; 32(2): 145–153.

4. Crary MA, Groher ME. Reinstituting oral feeding in tube-fed adult patients with dysphagia. *Nutr Clin Pract.* 2006; 21: 576–586.

5. Finestone, HM, Green-Finestone, LS. Rehabilitation medicine: 2. Diagnosis of dysphagia and its nutritional management for stroke patients. *CMAJ.* 2003; 169: 1041–1044.

6. Scolapio JS, Romano M, Neschia JF, Tarrosa V, Chukwudelunzu FE. PEG feeding tube placement following a stroke: when to place, when to wait. *Nutr Clin Pract.* 2000; 15: 36–39.

7. American Speech-Language Hearing Association Guidelines. *Clinical Indicators for Instrumental Assessment of Dysphagia. Special interest division 13, swallowing and swallowing disorders task force on clinical indicators* (2000). Accessed April 19, 2011, from http://www.asha.org/docs/pdf/GL2000-00047 .pdf

8. MedlinePlus. Bethesda, MD: U.S. National Library of Medicine (NLM); 2010. http://www.nlm.nih.gov/medlineplus/

9. Weekes E, Elia M. Resting energy expenditure and body composition following cerebro-vascular accident. *Clin Nutr.* 1992; 11(1): 18–22.

10. Ray S, Rana P, Rajput M, Haleem M. Nutritional management of stroke: from current evidence to conjecture. *Nutr Bull.* 2007; 32: 145–153.

11. Cook AM, Hatton J. Neurological Impairment. In: Gottschlich M, ed. *The A.S.P.E.N. Nutrition Support Core Curriculum.* Silver Spring, MD: American Society for Parenteral and Enteral Nutrition; 2007; 424–439.

12. Mike LA. Propofol-related infusion syndrome. *Practical Gastroenterology.* 2010:19–24.

13. Enteral Nutrition Board of Directors and Practice Recommendations Task Force: Bankhead R, Boullata J, Brantley S, et al. Enteral nutrition practice recommendations. *JPEN J Parenter Enteral Nutr.* 2009; 33:2, 122–167.

14. Corrigan ML, Escuro AA, Celestin J, Kirby DF. Nutrition in the Stroke Patient. *Nutr Clin Pract.* 2011; 26:3, 242–252.

15. Palmer J, Drennan JC, Baba M. Evaluation and treatment of swallowing impairments. *Am Fam Physician.* 2000; 61: 2453–2462.

16. McCallum, S. The National Dysphagia Diet: Implementation at a regional rehabilitation center and hospital system. *J Am Diet Assoc.* 2003; 103(3): 381–384.

17. American Dietetic Association (ADA): *International Dietetics & Nutrition Terminology (IDNT) Reference Manual: Standardized Language for the Nutrition Care Process*, 3rd ed. Chicago: ADA; 2010.

18. Heiss CJ, Goldberg L, Dzarnoski M. Registered dietitians and speech-language pathologists: an important partnership in dysphagia management. *J Am Diet Assoc.* 2010; 110(9): 1290–1293.

Endocrine and Renal Disease

Advanced Dietary Management in Type 1 Diabetes

LEARNING OBJECTIVES

Upon completing this case study, readers will be able to:

1. Describe how insulin management can be personalized for individual clients.
2. Outline methods for carbohydrate counting.
3. Identify types of insulin and their action curves.
4. Calculate typical carbohydrate: insulin ratios and insulin sensitivity factors.
5. Identify and manage symptoms of hypoglycemia.
6. Recognize the role of a Certified Diabetes Educator.

CASE DESCRIPTION/BACKGROUND

Type 1 diabetes is an insulin deficient state that results from pancreatic beta cell dysfunction. While the underlying cause of this disease remains unknown, it is thought that genetics and undetermined environmental factors contribute to an autoimmune destruction of the pancreatic beta cells. Type 1 diabetes typically presents during childhood and adolescence but can occur at any age (1).

When the body loses the ability to produce insulin, glucose transport into cells is impaired, and hyperglycemia results. Individuals with type 1 diabetes who do not produce insulin are at risk for diabetic ketoacidosis, a potentially fatal condition of hyperglycemia, accelerated ketone production, acid–base imbalance, and dehydration. Long-term complications of hyperglycemia include nephropathy, retinopathy, neuropathy, heart disease, and stroke. Exogenous insulin must be administered on a daily basis to control blood sugar and prevent both hyperglycemia and ketoacidosis. Insulin must be balanced with diet to promote normal blood sugars and prevent hypoglycemia (1,2).

The patient is a 30-year-old man with type 1 diabetes, diagnosed at age 13. He presents to the endocrinologist on 50 units of insulin glargine every evening and 3 units of lispro with each meal. His hemoglobin A1c (HbA1c) is elevated at 8.1% and he has experienced several instances of severe hypoglycemia in the last few months, the most recent causing loss of consciousness that resulted in his wife calling 9-1-1. He is seeking another opinion regarding his insulin regimen and diet.

During the first office visit, the endocrinologist determined that the client had no evidence of diabetes complications such as renal failure or cardiovascular disease. However, there was tremendous concern regarding the increased severity and frequency of the client's hypoglycemia. His glargine dose was decreased to 40 units. He was sent to the Registered Dietitian/Certified Diabetes Educator (RD/CDE) for diabetes education, as he had not received education since the time of his initial diagnosis.

Meal planning is a cornerstone of diabetes self-management and use of carbohydrate counting is one method of diabetes meal planning. *Carbohydrate counting* allows people who use rapid acting insulin before meals to fine-tune their pre-meal dose based upon the amount of carbohydrate they plan to eat. The RD/CDE introduced the concept of matching insulin to food intake and calculating insulin dose based upon the carbohydrate content of a meal or snack. She also recommended that he attend an insulin management program that would cover the concepts of (a) basal-prandial insulin; onset, peak, and duration of different types of insulin; and (b) proper storage and administration of insulin.

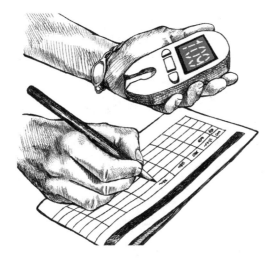

The RD/CDE helps him to determine his insulin: carbohydrate ratios, which will help him to know how much rapid acting insulin to administer at mealtimes. Two common methods are used for assigning carbohydrate ratios to a patient:

1. "500 Rule" where the insulin-to-carbohydrate ratio is derived by taking the total dose of all insulin taken in 24 hours, and dividing it into 500 (3). The result would usually be rounded to the nearest whole number.
2. It is also common to start with a ratio of 1 unit of insulin to every 15 grams of carbohydrate, and adjust upward or downward after observing 2-hour post-prandial and pre-meal blood glucose values for several days.

Once the carbohydrate-to-insulin ratio is determined, the patient counts carbohydrate grams for each meal, and then administers the appropriate prandial dose of insulin to cover the meal.

The RD/CDE also teaches him how to determine an insulin sensitivity factor, which helps to determine the dose of insulin that will "correct" a high blood sugar. Two methods are generally used to assign insulin sensitivity factors to a patient:

1. "1800 Rule" derived by taking the total daily dose of all insulin and dividing it into 1800 (3).

2. Start with a sensitivity of 50 and adjust it upward or downward after observing blood glucose levels for several days. In this case, 1 unit of insulin would be expected to drop the blood sugar by 50 units.

Using this method, if the blood sugar is high before a meal, the correction dose is added to the prandial dose.

Of note, the insulin sensitivity is typically 3 to 4 times the carbohydrate ratio. Patients may have different carbohydrate ratios and sensitivities at different times of the day. Generally, approximately 40% to 50% of insulin requirements are given as basal insulin and the remainder is divided up at mealtimes and snacks (3).

NUTRITIONAL ASSESSMENT DATA

1. Anthropometric Measurements.

Height: 5'11"
Weight: 175 lbs
BMI: 24.4

2. Biochemical Data.

Parameter	Value	Normal Range/Target* (may vary by age, sex, and lab)
Glucose	195 mg/dL	70–110 mg/dL
Hemoglobin A1c	8.1%	< 7%
Total cholesterol	152 mg/dL	< 200 mg/dL
LDL-cholesterol	79 mg/dL	< 100 mg/dL
HDL-cholesterol	62 mg/dL	> 40 mg/dL men > 50 mg/dL women
Triglycerides	87 mg/dL	< 150 mg/dL
Creatinine	0.8 mg/dL	0.7–1.4 mg/dL
TSH	1.80 mIU/L	0.40–4.50 IU/L

*Data from American Diabetes Association. Standards of Medical Care in Diabetes – 2010. *Diabetes Care*. 2010; 33(Suppl 1):511–561.

3. Nutrition-Focused Physical Findings.

BP: 110/70 mm/Hg

Abdominal exam reveals two areas of scar tissue to the right and left of
the umbilicus.

4. Client History.

The client is married without children. He works as a manager in a
busy office.

5. Food/Nutrition-Related History.

The RD/CDE gathered the following information:

Typically eats 3 meals and 1–2 snacks daily

Breakfast is usually around 7 AM; he sleeps later on weekends but
often has a low blood sugar if he sleeps too late.

Lunchtime can be quite variable due to work commitments and
at times he does not have an opportunity to eat until 2 PM
or later. He always experiences a low blood sugar when this
occurs.

Consumes fruit or pretzels in the car on the way home because of fear
of hypoglycemia while driving.

Dinner is typically at 7 or 8 PM; he often orders out.

If dinner is not late then he will have a snack before bedtime. He does
not take Lispro with his snacks.

Checks blood glucose (BG) 6 to 9 times a day. Takes insulin glargine
at bedtime which varies from 10 PM to 2 AM. Experiences 2 to 4
low blood sugars a week, often < 50 mg/dL; symptoms seem to
come on quickly and unexpectedly.

Relatively active: plays racquetball, basketball; regularly does yard
work and occasionally runs.

Uses alcohol socially 1 to 2 times a week.

Treats hypoglycemia with regular soda, candy, or "whatever is
around."

Typical food intake and blood sugar records with carbohydrate
counting:

Food Intake	Blood Sugar Level	Carbohydrate, g
Pre-breakfast	62	
Breakfast		
Cereal – 2 cups		74
Milk – 1.5 cups		18
Banana, small		20
Total carbohydrates		112
Two hours after breakfast	356	
Pre-lunch	105	
Lunch		
Tuna salad sandwich		30
1 oz bag of chips		16
1 apple		20
Total carbohydrates		66
Two hours post-lunch	210	
Snack		
1 oz bag of pretzels		22
1 peach		15
Total carbohydrates		37
Pre-dinner	250	
Dinner		
Frozen pizza, 2 slices		53
2 cups salad with oil and vinegar dressing		10
Total carbohydrate		63
Snack		
Large dish of ice cream (1½ cups)		50
Bedtime	298	

Review of food records also shows that while breakfast is fairly consistent on workdays, there is tremendous variability in the other meals and snacks from day to day.

Medications

Insulin glargine, 40 units every evening
Insulin lispro, 3 units with each meal (breakfast, lunch, and dinner)

QUESTIONS

1. Describe the management of blood glucose through intensive insulin therapy including self-monitoring of blood glucose (SMBG) and multiple daily injections of insulin (MDI). What are the advantages and disadvantages of this approach?
2. What is meant by basal–prandial insulin? What is the difference between the onset, peak, and duration of rapid-acting insulin analogs such as lispro, aspart, or glulisine and extended-acting insulin analogs such as glargine or detemir?
3. What is considered an optimal HbA1c level for a diabetic patient? What are the goals for preprandial and peak postprandial blood glucose levels?
4. Describe typical methods for teaching carbohydrate counting. How would an individual's level of motivation and education affect your choice of method to use?
5. Calculate a starting insulin-to-carbohydrate ratio based on his carbohydrate intake and insulin usage. Show your work. Based on his carbohydrate intake and blood sugar levels, what would the Certified Diabetes Educator recommend regarding his basal and prandial insulin dosages?
6. If his blood sugar were high in the morning or before a meal, how would the correction dose of insulin be determined? This is also known as the *insulin sensitivity factor*.
7. What are signs and symptoms of hypoglycemia? How would you recommend that he treats his hypoglycemia? Give specific suggestions.
8. What advice should he be given regarding his injection sites? Explain.
9. Discuss the role of the RD/CDE. What qualifications are necessary to become a Certified Diabetes Educator?
10. Write a PES statement for this patient upon presentation. What are your goals for this patient? How would you monitor the outcome (results) of his dietary treatment?

REFERENCES AND SUGGESTED READINGS

1. American Diabetes Association (ADA). Diagnosis and classification of diabetes mellitus. *Diabetes Care.* 2010; 33(Suppl 1):s62–s69.

2. American Diabetes Association (ADA). Nutrition recommendations and interventions for diabetes. *Diabetes Care.* 2008; 31(Suppl 1):s61–s78.

3. American Diabetes Association (ADA). *Getting Started with an Insulin Pump.* Accessed April 20, 2011 from http://www.diabetes.org/living-with-diabetes/ treatment-and-care/medication/insulin/getting-started.html

4. American Diabetes Association Standards of Medical Care in Diabetes – 2010. *Diabetes Care.* 2010; 33(Suppl 1):S511–S561.

5. Mayo Clinic. *Intensive Insulin Therapy: Achieving Tight Blood Sugar Control* (updated December 2010). Accessed April 20, 2011, from http://www .mayoclinic.com/health/intensive-insulin-therapy/DA00088

6. Herbold NH, Edelstein S. *Dietitian's Pocket Guide to Nutrition.* Sudbury, MA: Jones and Bartlett Publishers; 2010: 112.

7. American Dietetic Association (ADA), *International Dietetics & Nutrition Terminology (IDNT) Reference Manual: Standardized Language for the Nutrition Care Process*, 3rd ed. Chicago, IL: ADA; 2010.

Type 2 Diabetes in an Elderly Man

LEARNING OBJECTIVES

Upon completing this case study, readers will be able to:

1. Explain the pathophysiology of type 2 diabetes.
2. Evaluate dietary carbohydrate quantity and distribution in a diet record.
3. Identify the relationship between glycosylated hemoglobin levels and glycemic control.
4. Suggest an appropriate diet for a client with type 2 diabetes.

CASE DESCRIPTION/BACKGROUND

Over 25 million people in the United States have diabetes, with type 2 diabetes accounting for 90%–95% of known cases (1,2). Type 2 diabetes occurs when the cells of the body become resistant to insulin. These patients may have normal or even high levels of insulin but go on to develop hyperglycemia (2). Onset of type 2 diabetes is gradual, and is more likely to occur in older, obese, and sedentary patients as well as those with a family history of type 2 diabetes or a past history of gestational diabetes. The incidence is higher in some racial/ethnic groups including African Americans, Hispanic/Latino Americans, and American Indians.

Patients with type 2 diabetes are often treated with both diet and medications; some patients can control blood sugars with diet and lifestyle changes alone. Typical medications for type II diabetics work by increasing pancreatic insulin production, decreasing hepatic production of glucose, increasing the sensitivity of peripheral tissues to insulin, or inhibiting the absorption of dietary carbohydrate (3,4). Eventually the body may lose the ability to produce insulin, and exogenous insulin will be required. Regardless of the type of treatment for diabetes, diet therapy is an important facet of management. Matching dietary carbohydrate to the body's need can minimize fluctuations in blood sugars and help to prevent complications (5).

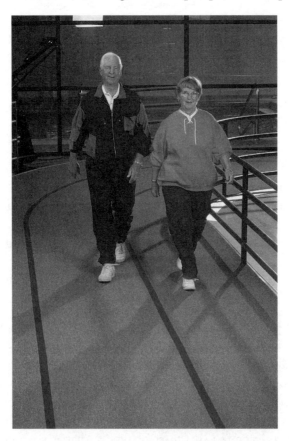

The client is a 73-year-old man diagnosed one year ago with type 2 diabetes mellitus. He has a history of coronary heart disease s/p angioplasty 5 years prior, hypertension, retinopathy, and left foot neuropathy. He makes every attempt to follow a healthy diet, and has been avoiding table sugar for the past year on his physician's advice. He comes to see the registered dietitian due to a persistently elevated hemoglobin A1c.

NUTRITIONAL ASSESSMENT DATA

1. Anthropometric Measurements.

Height: 6'2"
Weight 220 lbs

He weighed 240 lbs 5 years ago, and lost 30 pounds after his angioplasty by adopting a lower fat diet. He has since regained 10 pounds.

2. Biochemical Data.

Electrolytes, BUN, and creatinine values were normal.

Parameter	Value	Normal Range/Target* (may vary by age, sex, and lab)
Glucose (mid-morning fingerstick)	223 mg/dL	< 180 mg/dL after meals
Hemoglobin A1C	7.8%	< 7% in diabetes
Total cholesterol	160 mg/dL	< 200 mg/dL
LDL cholesterol	97 mg/dL	< 100 mg/dL
HDL cholesterol	55 mg/dL	> 40 mg/dL men > 50 mg/dL women
Triglycerides	87 mg/dL	< 150 mg/dL

*Data from American Diabetes Association. Standards of Medical Care in Diabetes – 2010. *Diabetes Care.* 2010; 33(Suppl 1):S511–S561.

3. Nutrition-Focused Physical Findings.

Blood pressure: 130/80 mm Hg.

4. Client History.

Family Hx

Paternal history is positive for heart disease and type 2 diabetes. He lives with his wife who does most of the cooking and shopping. He does not smoke and drinks alcohol socially. He gets little physical activity.

5. Food/Nutrition-Related History.

The following represents his usual intake.

Meal	Description
Breakfast	Cold cereal (raisin bran), 2 oz Nonfat milk, 1 cup Cranberry juice, 1 cup 2 slices rye toast with 2 tbs fruit spread Coffee with 2 tbs fat-free hazelnut creamer
Lunch	Turkey club sandwich: 3 oz turkey 1 tbs reduced fat mayonaise lettuce and tomato ¼ sliced avocado 2 slices turkey bacon 2 slices white bread, toasted Fresh fruit, 1 piece Tea with 1 tbs honey
Snack	2 fat-free fig cookies ½ cup apple cider
Dinner	6 oz fish or chicken, baked or broiled ½ cup cooked white rice or potato ½ cup cooked vegetable (carrots or green beans) 1 oz roll with 1 tbs stanol–ester enriched margarine Green salad with 2 tbs olive oil and 1 tbs vinegar Plain seltzer water, 12 oz
Evening snack	6 oz nonfat vanilla yogurt ¼ cup mixed nuts

Medications

Lipitor, Prevacid, ACTOplus met, and Januvia.

Supplements

No vitamins or supplements

QUESTIONS

1. What is his IBW, % IBW, and BMI? Estimate caloric requirements to promote an optimal weight.

2. Suggest an appropriate diet for him. What percent of his diet should come from carbohydrate? How many grams of carbohydrate should he have in a day? How should the carbohydrate be spread out over the day?

3. How does his current intake compare to his needs? Analyze his current intake and show your work. Approximately how many grams of carbohydrate is he currently consuming at each meal and snack? How do you think his low-fat diet has influenced his carbohydrate intake?

4. How do hemoglobin A1c levels correlate with blood sugar (mean plasma glucose) levels? Calculate his estimated average glucose based on his hemoglobin A1c levels. What factor(s) in his diet might be leading to his inability to further reduce his hemoglobin A1c, and what can you do to help him?

5. Explain the pathophysiology of type 2 diabetes. What risk factors does this client have for developing this condition?

6. What are the complications of type 2 diabetes? Which complications is he already experiencing? How can the dietitian assist in the management of type 2 diabetes and its associated problems?

7. Make a chart of common classes of oral medications for type 2 diabetes and how they are intended to work. Which ones is this client taking?

8. Identify an appropriate nutrition diagnosis and write a PES statement based on the available nutritional assessment data.

9. What are your goals for this client? How will you help him to achieve those goals, and what outcome measure(s) will you monitor to see that your intervention is working?

10. Write a note that documents your interaction with the patient using the SOAP or ADIME format.

REFERENCES AND SUGGESTED READINGS

1. U. S. Department of Health and Human Services (DHHS), Centers for Disease Control and Prevention (CDC). *National Diabetes Fact Sheet: National Estimates and General Information on Diabetes and Prediabetes in the United States, 2011.* Accessed April 20, 2011, from http://www.cdc.gov/diabetes/pubs/pdf/ndfs_2011.pdf

2. American Diabetes Association (ADA). Diagnosis and classification of diabetes mellitus. *Diabetes Care.* 2010; 33(Suppl 1):S62–S69.

3. Sonnenberg GE, Kotchen TA. New therapeutic approaches to reversing insulin resistance. *Curr Opin NephrolHypertens.* 1998; 7(5):551–556.
4. Medications. American Diabetes Association (ADA). Accessed April 20, 2011, from http://www.diabetes.org/type-2-diabetes/oral-medications.jsp
5. American Diabetes Association (ADA). Nutrition recommendations and interventions for diabetes: a position statement of the American Diabetes Association. *Diabetes Care.* 2008; 31(Suppl 1):S61–S78.
6. Sheard NF, Clark NG, Brand-Miller JC, et al. Dietary carbohydrate (amount and type) in the prevention and management of diabetes. *Diabetes Care.* 2004; 27(9):2266–2271.
7. Nathan DM, Kuenen J, Borg R, Zheng H, Schoenfeld D, Heine R. Translating the A1c assay into estimated average glucose values. *Diabetes Care.* 2008; 31(1):1–6.
8. American Dietetic Association (ADA), *International Dietetics & Nutrition Terminology (IDNT) Reference Manual: Standardized Language for the Nutrition Care Process,* 3rd ed. Chicago, IL: ADA; 2010.

14

Polycystic Ovary Syndrome in a Young Woman

LEARNING OBJECTIVES

Upon completing this case study, readers will be able to:

1. Describe polycystic ovary syndrome and its associated risks.
2. Assess the nutritional status of a patient with polycystic ovary syndrome.
3. Explain the relationship between diet and insulin resistance.
4. Suggest appropriate dietary interventions for a patient with polycystic ovary syndrome.
5. Identify goals of therapy and outcomes for monitoring and evaluation of a patient with polycystic ovary syndrome.

CASE DESCRIPTION/BACKGROUND

Polycystic ovary syndrome (PCOS) affects 10% of women in the United States and is the most common cause of menstrual irregularities and infertility (1). PCOS has been viewed as a collection of reproductive health problems characterized by oligo- or anovulation, high levels of androgen hormones, and polycystic ovaries. Symptoms include infrequent and/or irregular periods, infertility, and miscarriage associated with androgenic symptoms such as hirsutism, acne, and male-pattern hair loss (2,3). Although the exact cause of PCOS is unknown, insulin is thought to play a central role in the pathophysiology (3,4). Many women with PCOS are insulin resistant: the resulting hyperinsulinemia stimulates ovarian insulin receptors, which in turn causes the ovaries to produce greater-than-normal amounts of testosterone. The testosterone, in turn, inhibits ovulation and causes the androgenic symptoms (5).

PCOS is often accompanied by overweight or obesity, dyslipidemia, hypertension, and metabolic syndrome (3,4). Diet and physical activity are the primary treatment approaches for managing PCOS and these associated conditions (6–8). Insulin-sensitizers may be used in conjunction with lifestyle modification (9). Dietary guidelines include a reduced carbohydrate diet with an emphasis on whole grains, lean proteins, and omega-3 fatty acids (10,11).

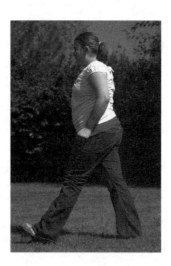

The client is a 27-year-old woman who was diagnosed with PCOS four years ago. She has a history of irregular menstrual periods, occurring every 3 to 4 months and lasting 6 days, on average. She is insulin resistant. The client had been prescribed metformin, although she confessed that she was "sporadic" in taking her medications.

She lives with her grandmother who has type 2 diabetes. The client does most of the cooking. The client comes to the registered dietitian to lose weight and reduce her risk for developing diabetes.

NUTRITIONAL ASSESSMENT DATA

1. Anthropometric Measurements.

Height: 5'7"
Weight: 225 lbs

2. Biochemical Data.

Parameter	Value	Normal Values* (may vary by age, sex, and lab)
Insulin (fasting)	22.4	2–20 µU/mL
Testosterone	82	6–86 ng/dL (female)
HbA1c	5.9	4.0%–6.0%
Glucose (fasting)	97	70–110 mg/dL
Total cholesterol	207	< 200 mg/dL
LDL cholesterol	100	< 100 mg/dL
Triglycerides	230	< 150 mg/dL

*Data from Morris JC. *Dietitian's Guide to Assessment and Documentation.* Sudbury, MA: Jones & Bartlett Learning; 2011.
Kratz A, Ferraro M, Sluss PM, Lewandrowski KB. Laboratory reference values. N Engl J Med. 2004; 351:1548–1563.

3. Nutrition-Focused Physical Findings.

Vital Signs

Blood pressure: 118/75 mm/Hg

Observations

The patient has excess facial hair on her upper lip and chin; balding; acanthosis nigricans on back of neck; skin tags on neck; excess weight in abdominal area; acne on face.

4. Client History.

Social Hx

Single woman, lives with and cares for her grandmother. Has a government job in the city. She is inactive but has a gym membership. She likes to dance. The client does not smoke. She does not drink alcohol.

5. Food/Nutrition-Related History.

The following represents her usual intake:

Meal	Time	Description
Breakfast	8 AM	1 soft pretzel with mustard or a plain bagel with butter
Lunch	12 PM	Hamburger or meatball sandwich 16 oz juice small bag of chips or a side of soup (chicken noodle)
Snack	3 PM	1 cup tea with 1 tbs sugar (she does not like sugar substitutes)
Dinner	5:30 PM	Grilled steak, approximately 8 oz Garden salad with 2 tbs ranch dressing Two biscuits with 1 tsp butter each 16 oz juice
Snack	8 PM	1 cup pretzels 8 oz juice

Medications

2,000 mg metformin

Supplements

None

QUESTIONS

1. Define polycystic ovary syndrome.
2. What signs and symptoms of PCOS does the patient have? Discuss how PCOS affects her risk for future health problems.
3. What are the diet recommendations for someone with PCOS?
4. Analyze her diet for kilocalories, protein, fat, saturated fat, carbohydrate, fiber, and sodium. Show your work.
5. How does her diet compare to the recommendations in question #3? Justify your answer by comparing intake to recommended levels.
6. What type of medication is metformin, and how does it work? Are there any side effects?

7. Suggest specific modifications of diet and lifestyle (interventions) that might improve this patient's health.
8. Write a PES statement that would apply to this patient.
9. What are your overall goals for this client, and how would you monitor the effectiveness of your interventions?
10. Write a note in ADIME or SOAP format that summarizes your assessment.

REFERENCES AND SUGGESTED READINGS

1. Azziz R, Woods KS, Reyna R, et al. The prevalence and features of polycystic ovary syndrome in an unselected population. *J Clin Endocrinol Metab.* 2004; 89:2745–2749.
2. Balen A, Michelmore K. What is polycystic ovary syndrome? *Hum Reprod.* 2002; 17(9): 2219–2227.
3. Setji TL, Brown AJ. Polycystic ovary syndrome: Diagnosis and treatment. *Am J Med,* 2007; 120:128-132.
4. Norman RJ, Dewailly D, Legro RS, Hickey TE. Polycystic ovary syndrome. *Lancet,* 2007; 370: 685–697.
5. Sherif K. Understanding PCOS. In: Grassi A, ed. *The Dietitian's Guide to Polycystic Ovary Syndrome.* Luca Publishing: Haverford, PA; 2007.
6. Grassi A. Dietary strategies and lifestyle modification for polycystic ovary syndrome. In: Grassi A, ed. *The Dietitian's Guide to Polycystic Ovary Syndrome.* Luca Publishing, Haverford, PA; 2007: 35–62.
7. Moran LJ, Brinkworth G, Noakes M, Norman RJ. Effects of lifestyle modification in polycystic ovarian syndrome. *Reprod Biomed Online.* 2006; 12:569–578.
8. Pasquali R. Role of changes in dietary habits in polycystic ovary syndrome. *Reprod BioMed Online.* 2004; 8(4):431–439.
9. Sharma S, Nestler J. Prevention of diabetes and cardiovascular disease in women with PCOS: treatment with insulin sensitizers. *Best Practice Research Clin Endo Metab.* 2006; 20(2):245–260.
10. Marsh K, Brand-Miller J. The optimal diet for women with polycystic ovary syndrome. *Br J Nutr.* 2005; 94:154–165.
11. Grassi A. Practical applications: Medical nutrition therapy and the role of the dietitian in the treatment of polycystic ovary syndrome. In: Grassi A, ed. *The Dietitian's Guide to Polycystic Ovary Syndrome.* Luca Publishing, Haverford, PA; 2007: 63–92.
12. Marsh KA, Steinbeck KS, Atkinson FS, Petocz P, Brand-Miller JC. Effect of a low glycemic index compared with a conventional healthy diet on polycystic ovary syndrome. *Am J Clin Nutr.* 2010; 92:83–92.

13. The Rotterdam ESHRE/ASRM sponsored PCOS consensus workshop group: revised 2003 consensus on diagnostic criteria and long term health risks related to polycystic ovary syndrome. *Fertil Steril.* 2004; 81:19–25.
14. Palomba S, Falbo S, Zullo F, Orio F Jr. Evidence-based and potential benefits of metformin in the polycystic ovary syndrome: a comprehensive review. *Endocr Rev.* 2009; 30:1–50.
15. American Dietetic Association (ADA). *International Dietetics & Nutrition Terminology (IDNT) Reference Manual: Standardized Language for the Nutrition Care Process,* 3rd ed. Chicago, IL: ADA; 2010.

Chronic Kidney Disease: Nutrition for Hemodialysis

LEARNING OBJECTIVES

Upon completing this case study, readers will be able to:

1. Assess the nutritional status of a patient with chronic kidney disease (CKD).
2. Describe the pathophysiology of chronic renal failure (CRF).
3. Determine an appropriate nutrient prescription for an individual with Stage 5 CKD.
4. Recommend changes to usual dietary intake that will help to achieve acceptable metabolic parameters in a CKD patient.
5. Discuss methods of controlling phosphate levels in this population.
6. Identify goals of diet therapy and outcomes for monitoring and evaluation of a patient with CKD.

CASE DESCRIPTION/BACKGROUND

Chronic kidney disease (CKD) is defined as a progressive decline in kidney function for three months or more as measured by glomerular filtration rate (GFR) (1). Normal kidney functions include filtration of waste products, fluid and electrolyte regulation, and endocrine functions including production of renin, erythropoietin, and calcitriol. CKD is classified into five stages based on GFR, which is a calculated value based on data including serum creatinine, age, gender, and race (1). Stage 1 CKD is defined as kidney damage with normal or increased GFR. Stages 2–4 are marked by a progressive decline in GFR. At Stage 5, renal replacement therapy (RRT) such as hemodialysis, peritoneal dialysis, or kidney transplant is required to sustain life (1,2).

Kidney disease affects the intake, absorption, metabolism, and excretion of various nutrients, including protein, energy, sodium, potassium, calcium, phosphorus, vitamin D, and iron (2–4). Protein energy malnutrition often develops over the course of the disease and is correlated with poor outcomes. It is important that clients with chronic kidney disease receive nutritional assessment, dietary modification, counseling, and follow up from a registered dietitian (2–4).

The client is an 81-year-old African-American man with a history of hypertension, coronary artery disease, mitral valve disorder, heart failure, benign prostatic hypertrophy, and gout. He has stage 5 CKD and was recently started on hemodialysis three times weekly for 4 hours per treatment. The dialysate is a standard formula with a 2.0 potassium, 2.0 calcium composition. He is oliguric with a residual urine output of 500 mL or less per day.

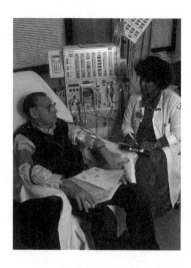

NUTRITIONAL ASSESSMENT DATA

1. Anthropometric Measurements.

Height: 5'9"
Weight: 143 lbs post-dialysis; 153 lbs predialysis
Usual weight: 170–175 lbs
Weight change: Lost 30 lbs in past year

2. Biochemical Data.

Values are pre-dialysis treatment.

Parameter	Value	Normal Range * (may vary by age, sex, and lab)	
Sodium	141 mEq/L	135–147 mEq/L	
Potassium	5.9 mEq/L	3.5–5.0 mEq/L	H
Chloride	103 mEq/L	98–106 mEq/L	
Carbon dioxide	22 mEq/L	21–30 mEq/L	
BUN	68 mg/dL	8–23 mg/dL	H
Creatinine	7.1 mg/dL	0.7–1.5 mg/dL	H
Glomerular filtration rate	10 mL/min/1.73 m^2	90–120 mL/min/1.73 m^2	L
Glucose	99 mg/dL	70–110 mg/dL	
Hemoglobin	12.2 g/dL	14–18 g/dL (men)	L
Hematocrit	41.8%	38–54 % (men)	
Albumin	3.7 g/dL	3.5–5.5 g/dL	
Phosphorus	8.4 mg/dL	3.0–4.5 mg/dL	H
Calcium	9.6 mg/dL	9–11 mg/dL	
Corrected calcium	9.8 mg/dL	9–11 mg/dL	
PTH – intact	147 mmol/L	150–300 mmol/L in dialysis patients	L

*Data from U. S. Food and Drug Administration (FDA). *Investigations Operations Manual.* Silver Spring, MD: US FDA; 2001. Accessed April 21, 2011, from http://www.fda.gov/downloads/ICECI/Inspections/IOM/UCM135835.pdf

Morris JC. *Dietitian's Guide to Assessment and Documentation.* Sudbury, MA: Jones & Bartlett Learning; 2011.

National Kidney Foundation (NKF). K/DOQI clinical practice guidelines for bone metabolism and disease in chronic kidney disease. *Am J Kidney Dis.* 2003; 42(Suppl 3):S1–S202.

3. Nutrition-Focused Physical Findings.

The patient appears oriented but does seem lethargic at times. His oral health is good and he has his own teeth. He appears to have some wasting of muscle and fat stores due to weight loss. He is mentally alert.

4. Client History.

Social Hx

History of smoking and alcohol use, none currently. He and his wife show interest in his care and are receptive to dietary counseling. His wife is responsible for food shopping and meal preparation.

5. Food/Nutrition-Related History.

The registered dietitian takes a 24-hour recall from the patient.

Breakfast

    1 hard-boiled egg
    ½ cup raisin bran with 1 cup 2% milk
    2 pancakes, maple syrup
    12-oz mug of coffee with cream and sugar

Lunch

    ham sandwich (approximately 2 oz of ham on whole wheat bread)
        with lettuce and 1 tsp mayonnaise
    ½ cup Jello
    8 oz glass of apple juice

Dinner

    fried chicken thigh
    small portions of canned string beans and corn
    ½ cup cantaloupe
    corn muffin with 1 tsp margarine
    12 oz can of diet cola

Snacks, afternoon and evening

    2 oz dry roasted, salted peanuts
    4 chocolate wafer cookies
    16 oz water

When his wife left the room for a moment, he also admitted to sneaking an extra 12 oz can of diet cola.

Medications

Oral: calcium acetate 667 mg, 2 tabs with meals TID, warfarin 3 mg, valsartan 160 mg, carvedilol 3.125 mg, colchicine 0.6 mg prn, aspirin 81 mg, allopurinol 100 mg.

IV: iron sucrose 100 mg every 2 weeks, epoetin alpha 11,600 units every treatment, paricalcitol 6 mcg every treatment.

Supplements

None.

QUESTIONS

1. Calculate his BMI and % UBW. Why was his weight taken before and after dialysis? Which of those values should you used to calculate the BMI and % UBW? Comment on his nutritional status.

2. Calculate his needs for calories and protein. Show your work. How much sodium, potassium, and phosphorus should he have on a daily basis? Explain why these nutrients need to be limited.

3. What do the terms *anuric* and *oliguric* mean? Since the patient is oliguric, how much fluid should he take in daily? Is his fluid intake too low, too high, or just right? In addition to his reported intake, how would you know if he were drinking the right amount of fluid between dialysis treatments? What is an expected fluid weight gain between dialysis treatments? What are the potential consequences for drinking too much fluid?

4. Explain what the corrected calcium × phosphorus (Ca × P) product is, and why it matters. Calculate his corrected Ca × P product. What medication is he currently on to bind his phosphorus? What changes could you suggest to bring his Ca × P product closer to desired values?

5. Explain why patients with kidney failure become anemic. Identify the medications that he is on to address his anemia.

6. What is secondary hyperparathyroidism (HPT), and why does it occur in chronic kidney disease? How is secondary HPT

commonly treated? What medication is he on to help with this condition?

7. Analyze his current intake for kcals, protein, sodium, potassium, and phosphorus using the USDA database or a standard nutritional analysis program that includes phosphorus. Show your work. How does his intake compare to his needs for these nutrients? Rewrite a sample diet for him based on his usual intake. Make sure that the new diet meets his kcal and protein needs without exceeding limits on sodium, potassium, phosphorus, or fluid. Show your work by including a table or report with food choices and nutrient levels.

8. Should he take a renal multivitamin? What is the difference between a renal multivitamin and a standard multivitamin?

9. Choose a Nutrition Diagnosis and write a PES statement.

10. What are your goals for nutrition therapy? Specify how you would monitor outcomes for this patient.

REFERENCES AND SUGGESTED READINGS

1. National Kidney Foundation. K/DOQI clinical practice guidelines for chronic kidney disease: evaluation, classification, and stratification. *Am J Kidney Dis.* 2002; 39(2 Suppl 1): S1–S266.

2. National Kidney Foundation (NKF). K/DOQI nutrition in chronic renal failure. *Am J Kidney Dis.* 2000; 35:6(Suppl 2):S1–S139.

3. Beto JA, Bansal VK. Medical nutrition therapy in chronic kidney failure: integrating clinical practice guidelines. *J Am Diet Assoc* 2004; 104:404–409.

4. Thomas R, Kanso A, Sedor JR. Chronic kidney disease and its complications. *Prim Care Clin Office Pract.* 2008; 35:329–344.

5. Kent PS. Integrating clinical nutrition practice guidelines in chronic kidney disease. *Nutr Clin Pract.* 2005; 20:213–217.

6. Nanovic L. Electrolyte and fluid management in hemodialysis and peritoneal dialysis. *Nutr Clin Pract.* 2005; 20:192–201.

7. National Kidney Foundation (NKF). K/DOQI clinical practice guidelines for bone metabolism and disease in chronic kidney disease. *Am J Kidney Dis.* 2003; 42(4 Suppl 3):S1–S202.

8. Medline Plus. *Urine output - decreased.* Bethesda, MD: National Library of Medicine (NLM); September 30, 2009. Accessed January 8, 2011, from http://www.nlm.nih.gov/medlineplus/ency/article/003147.htm

9. Fouque D, Vennegoor M, Wee PT. EBPG guideline on nutrition. *Nephrol Dial Transplant.* 2007; 22(Suppl 2):ii45–ii87.

10. Nankivell BJ, Murali KM. Renal failure from vitamin C after transplantation. *N Engl J Med.* 2008; 358:4.

11. American Dietetic Association (ADA). *International Dietetics & Nutrition Terminology (IDNT) Reference Manual: Standardized Language for the Nutrition Care Process,* 3rd ed. Chicago, IL: ADA; 2010.

Oncology and Hematology

Pancreatic Cancer Status Post-Whipple Procedure

LEARNING OBJECTIVES

Upon completing this case study, readers will be able to:

1. Identify nutritional deficiencies associated with pancreatic cancer and its treatment.
2. Identify symptoms most commonly associated with pancreatic enzyme insufficiency.
3. Implement dietary interventions for maximum symptom management and nutritional repletion.
4. Identify goals of medical nutrition therapy for a patient with pancreatic cancer and outcomes for monitoring and evaluation of treatment.

CASE DESCRIPTION/BACKGROUND

Pancreatic cancer often develops without symptoms and is rarely detected early. According to the American Cancer Society (ACS), it was ranked number 10 in leading sites of new cancer cases, but number 4 in new cancer deaths in 2010 (1). 80%–90% of pancreatic cancer patients present with weight loss and malabsorption at the time of diagnosis (2). Pancreatic cancer can interfere with nutritional intake and absorption through several mechanisms. Physical effects of the tumor can cause gastric outlet obstruction with early satiety and emesis; obstruction of the pancreatic and common bile ducts leads to diminished availability of bile, bicarbonate, and pancreatic enzymes. Cancer cachexia with wasting and malnutrition is common in pancreatic cancer and may be related to tumor and proinflammatory cytokine activity (3). Furthermore, pancreatic tissue destruction results in decreased production of digestive enzymes and impairment of pancreatic exocrine function (2). Endocrine pancreatic function may also be affected in some cases and may be associated with diabetes (3).

Pancreatic cancer patients may suffer from gastrointestinal symptoms related to their disease as well as to the side effects of treatment. The treatment for pancreatic cancer may involve surgery, chemotherapy, and/or radiation therapy, all of which can alter nutritional status. The dietetic practitioner should be familiar with the anatomy and physiology of the pancreas, the pathophysiology after partial or total surgical resection, and the consequences of chemotherapy and radiation therapy in order to help manage nutritional deficiencies. Dietary modification and pancreatic enzyme replacement can help to alleviate malabsorption and gastrointestinal symptoms in pancreatic cancer (2–4).

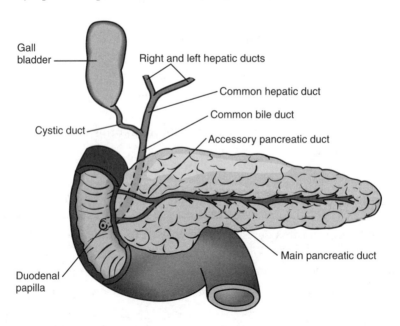

The client is a 56-year-old woman, a smoker with a past medical history of hypercholesterolemia and osteoporosis. Her initial presentation to the emergency room was for abdominal and low back pain, jaundice, and heartburn. Further examination and abdominal magnetic resonance imaging (MRI) revealed a 2 cm mass in the pancreas with distal bile duct obstruction. Ten days later, a Whipple procedure (pancreaticoduoenec-tomy) was performed. Post-op complications included pleural effusion, perihepatic abscess, DVT, and obstructive jaundice. Chemotherapy was initiated 3 months after her original presentation with gemcitabine HCl. By month 4, she was referred to the registered dietitian for evaluation due to weight loss. Over the next eight months, she continued to receive gemcitabine along with a course of fluorouracil and radiation therapy. During month 11, she suffered T12 and L2 compression fractures, for which she was treated with kyphoplasty.

NUTRITIONAL ASSESSMENT DATA

1. Anthropometric Measurements.

Height: 5'2" (or 62")
Weight:

Baseline	3 months	4 months	10 months
150 lb	135 lb	126 lb	125 lb

Weight trends are in Figure 16.1.

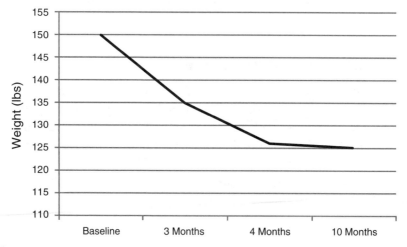

Figure 16.1 Weight Trends

2. Biochemical Data.

Parameter	Months 3	4	10	Units	Normal Range* (may vary by age, sex, and lab)
Hemoglobin	10.1	10.1	9.7	g/dL	12–16 g/dL (women)
Hematocrit	29.5	29.8	28.4	%	36%–47% (women)
White blood cells	12.2	8.2	2.4	cells × 10³/mm³	4.5–11.0 10³/mm³
Glucose	76	97	119	mg/dL	70–110 mg/dL
Albumin	3.0	3.4	3.1	g/dL	3.5–5.5 g/dL
Prealbumin	8	12	23	mg/dL	16–40 mg/dL
Sodium	141	138	140	mEq/L	135–147 mEq/L
Potassium	3.5	4.3	4.1	mEq/L	3.5–5.5 mEql/L
Chloride	105	102	104	mEq/L	98–106 mEq/L
Carbon dioxide	20	23	22	mEq/L	21–30 mEq/L
BUN	9	14	10	mg/dL	8–23 mg/dL
Creatinine	0.5	0.6	0.6	mg/dL	0.7–1.5 mg/dL
25 OH Vitamin D	–	< 7	19.3	ng/mL	32–100 ng/mL
C-reactive protein	–	0.3	–	mg/L	0.08–3.10 mg/L

*Data from U. S. Food and Drug Administration (FDA). *Investigations Operations Manual.* Silver Spring, MD: US FDA; 2001. Accessed April 21, 2011, from http://www.fda.gov/downloads/ICECI/Inspections/IOM/UCM135835.pdf
Morris JC. *Dietitian's Guide to Assessment and Documentation.* Sudbury, MA: Jones & Bartlett Learning; 2011.
Kratz A, Ferraro M, Sluss PM, Lewandrowski KB. Laboratory reference values. *N Engl J Med.* 2004; 351(15):1548–1563.

3. Nutrition-Focused Physical Findings.

The treating registered dietitian established a goal weight of 130 lb. A bioelectrical impedance analysis was conducted to assess body composition. The results revealed severe muscle wasting at 74% optimum (32 lb of lean muscle mass vs. 43 lb optimal). Measured body composition was 25% lean muscle mass, 36% fat and 38% extracellular tissue. Resting metabolic rate was measured using a hand held calorimeter at 1200 kilocalories daily.

4. Client History.

Social Hx

The client is married with no children. She currently smokes ½ pack of cigarettes per day. Drinks alcohol socially.

Family Hx

Her family history is unremarkable for cancer.

5. Food/Nutrition-Related History.

The client complained of weakness, pain, belching, gas, and severe cramping associated with meals. Her bowel movements were erratic and fluctuated between constipation and diarrhea. She also complained of dry mouth and taste changes. A 24-hour recall was obtained.

Usual Diet

Food	Amount Eaten	Tablets/Units of Lipase Taken
Breakfast		2 Tabs, 4000 units lipase each
French toast	1 slice	
Butter	1 pat	
Syrup	1 tbs	
Fruit Salad	½ cup	
Tea with sugar	1 cup tea, 1 tsp sugar	
Lunch		2 Tabs, 4000 units lipase each
Broiled salmon	2 oz	
Lentil soup	¾ cup	
Water	12 oz	
Snack		
Egg salad	¼ cup	
Crackers, butter type	5	
Unsweetened iced tea	8 oz	
Dinner		2 Tabs, 4000 units lipase each
Roast pork	2 oz	

(continues)

(Continued)

Food	Amount Eaten	Tablets/Units of Lipase Taken
Mashed potato made with butter	1/3 cup	
Gravy	2 tbs	
Applesauce	½ cup	
Water	12 oz	
Snack		
Ginger ale	8 oz	
Vanilla ice cream	½ cup	
Between meal supplements		
High protien oral nutritional supplement with 250 kcals, 11 g protien, 9 g fat/can	2.5 cans	

Medications

oxycodone, lansoprazole, teriparatide, pancrelipase (4000 units lipase, 25,000 units amylase, and 25,000 units protease per tablet)

Supplements

Vitamin D 200 IU plus calcium carbonate, 500 mg

QUESTIONS

1. Calculate her % UBW and BMI at months 3, 4, and 10. Comment on the trends in her weight and BMI. If a 5% weight loss in 1 month and 10% weight loss at 6 months indicates nutrition risk, what does her weight loss suggest?
2. Analyze her total calorie intake, including her protein and fat intake in grams. Show your work for each food item and subtotals for each meal.
3. Indirect calorimetry measured at resting metabolic rate of 1200 kcals per day. How is this number used to estimate total energy needs for the day? Compare the results to her food recall. Is she eating enough to meet her nutritional requirements? Why do you think she continues to lose weight?

4. Explain what a Whipple procedure is and describe postoperative nutrition-related complications. What are the main dietary interventions for patients who have had the procedure?

5. Describe signs and symptoms of pancreatic enzyme insufficiency. Identify signs from her history that may suggest pancreatic enzyme insufficiency. How are pancreatic enzymes typically dosed according to dietary fat intake? Based on your analysis of her meals, do you think that changes should be made in her enzyme therapy?

6. Identify symptoms in her history that may be side effects of the chemotherapy and discuss the intervention.

7. Why is it important to monitor her Vitamin D level? Explain the factors in her case that may contribute to a Vitamin D deficiency. Explain which test is used to assess Vitamin D levels, what the expected normal ranges are, and why it is important to have a normal Vitamin D level.

8. What other micronutrient deficiencies should you be concerned about?

9. Write a PES statement or statements based on the available nutritional assessment data from month 4.

10. What are your overall goals for this patient? Name the specific interventions that would address her nutrition diagnoses, and specify how you would monitor their effectiveness.

REFERENCES AND SUGGESTED READINGS

1. American Cancer Society (ACS). *Cancer Facts and Figures 2010*. Atlanta, GA: ACS; 2011. Accessed April 21, 2011, from http://www.cancer.org/Research/CancerFactsFigures/index

2. Damerla V, Gotlieb V, Larson H, Saif MW. Pancreatic enzyme supplementation in pancreatic cancer. *J Support Oncol.* 2008; 6:393–396.

3. Pappas S, Krzywda E, Mcdowell N. Nutrition and pancreaticoduodenectomy. *Nutr Clin Pract.* 2010; 25(3):234–243.

4. National Cancer Institute (NCI). *Pancreatic Cancer Treatment (PDQ®)*. Last modified 03/05/2010. Accessed April 21, 2011, from http://www.cancer.gov/cancertopics/pdq/treatment/pancreatic/HealthProfessional/page2

5. Frary CD, Johnson RK. Nutrition basics. In: Mahan LK, Escott-Stump S, eds. *Krause's Food & Nutrition Therapy,* 12 ed., St. Louis, MO: Saunders Elsevier; 2008: 22–38.

6. Delegge MH, Drake LM. Nutritional assessment. *Gastroenterology Clin N Am.* 2007; 36:1–22.

7. U.S. Department of Agriculture (USDA), Agricultural Research Service. *USDA National Nutrient Database for Standard Reference, Release 23* (2010). Nutrient Data Laboratory Home Page. Accessed April 21, 2011, from http://www.ars.usda.gov/nutrientdata

8. Pellet P. Food energy requirements in humans. *Am J Clin Nutr.* 1990; 51:711–722.

9. Petzel M, Meddles J. Medical nutrition therapy for patients with pancreatic cancer. *Oncology Nutrition Connection.* 2005; 2:15–18.

10. Pancreatic Cancer Action Network (PANCAN). Diet and nutrition: nutritional concerns with pancreatic cancer. Pancreatic Cancer Action Network (PANCAN) pamphlet. Manhattan Beach, CA: PACAN; 2007.

11. Appendix A. Tips for managing nutrition impact symptoms. In: Elliott L, Molseed L, McCallum P, eds. *The Clinical Guide to Oncology Nutrition*, 2nd ed. Chicago, IL: American Dietetic Association; 2006: 241–245.

12. Hollis B. Assessment and interpretation of circulating 25-hydroxyvitamin D and 1,25-dihydroxyvitamin D in the clinical environment. *Endocrinol Metab Clin N Am.* 2010; 39:271–286.

13. Thomas S. Nutritional implications of surgical oncology. In: Elliott L, Molseed L, McCallum P, eds. *The Clinical Guide to Oncology Nutrition*, 2nd ed. Chicago, IL: American Dietetic Association; 2006: 94–109.

14. American Dietetic Association (ADA). *International Dietetics & Nutrition Terminology (IDNT) Reference Manual: Standardized Language for the Nutrition Care Process*, 3rd ed. Chicago, IL: ADA; 2010.

17

Esophageal Cancer with Enteral Nutrition

LEARNING OBJECTIVES

Upon completing this case study, readers will be able to:

1. Assess nutritional status in a patient with esophageal cancer.
2. Determine nutritional requirements of a patient with esophageal cancer.
3. Predict possible nutrition-related side effects of chemotherapy and radiation.
4. Calculate an enteral feeding regimen to meet nutritional needs.

CASE DESCRIPTION/BACKGROUND

Esophageal cancer is the seventh leading cause of death worldwide, and has been on the rise in the United States over the past few decades (1,2). Nutritional management is complicated by difficulty with oral intake due to obstruction of the esophagus by the tumor. Most patients present with dysphagia and weight loss, symptoms which may not develop until after the disease has progressed to an advanced stage (2,3). Patients with esophageal cancer have been noted to have a higher percentage of weight loss than patients with other types of cancer, and malnutrition is common (3,4).

Dysphagia, cancer cachexia, and the effects of chemotherapy, radiation, and surgery all contribute to a unique challenge in maintaining adequate nutrition in this population. Many patients are treated with chemotherapy and radiation prior to surgery. A high protein, high calorie, consistency modified diet should be attempted during this time, but dysphagia and esophagitis caused by radiation may preclude adequate oral nutrition and hydration. Nutrition support may be needed during treatment both pre- and post-operatively (4,5). While the enteral route is preferred to parenteral, preoperative tube feeding presents a challenge with regard to enteral access. Percutaneous endoscopic gastrostomy (PEG) tubes and nasoenteric tubes may not be possible in esophageal cancer due to obstruction of the esophagus by the tumor. With a PEG tube, there is a risk of damage to the portion of the stomach or its blood supply, which will eventually be used as a conduit during esophagectomy, and the potential exists for spreading tumor cells during the PEG procedure (3-6). Laparoscopically placed feeding tubes may be an option preoperatively, and esophageal stents are sometimes used to facilitate oral intake (3,6). Jejunostomy tubes are frequently placed during the esophagectomy procedure, and can be used for post-operative nutrition support.

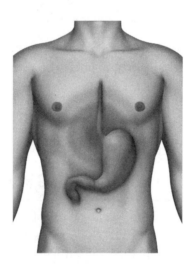

The patient is a 56-year-old man with a history of gastroesophageal reflux disease, Barrett's esophagus, and a 30 pack per year history of smoking. He presents with a two month history of coughing, sore throat, and progressive difficulty swallowing, first of solid foods and more recently of liquids. He is currently experiencing nausea and early satiety. A biopsy revealed adenocarcinoma of the distal esophagus and gastroesophageal junction. Following chemotherapy with 5-fluorouracil and cisplatin, along with radiation, an esophagectomy and j-tube placement are planned.

NUTRITIONAL ASSESSMENT DATA

1. Anthropometric Measurements.

Height: 5'8"
Weight: 165 lbs
Usual weight: 185 lbs (4 months ago)

2. Biochemical Data and Test Results.

Parameter	Result	Normal Range* (may vary by age, sex, and lab)	
Sodium	140 mEq/L	135–147 mEq/L	
Potassium	4.3 mEq/L	3.5–5.0 mEq/L	
Chloride	100 mEq/L	98–106 mEq/L	
CO_2	25 mEq/L	21–30 mEq/L	
BUN	15 mg/dL	8–23 mg/dL	
Creatinine	0.9 mg/dL	0.7–1.5 mg/dL	
Glucose	89 mg/dL	70–110 mg/dL	
Phosphorus	3.2 mg/dL	3.0–4.5 mg/dL	
Albumin	2.9 mg/dL	3.5–5.5 g/dL	L
Prealbumin	8 mg/dL	16–40 mg/dL	L
Hemoglobin	13.8 mg/dL	14–18 g/dL (men) 12–16 g/dL (women)	L
Hematocrit	37%	38–54% (men) 36–47% (women)	L

*Data from U. S. Food and Drug Administration (FDA). *Investigations Operations Manual.* Silver Spring, MD: US FDA; 2001. Accessed April 21, 2011, from http://www.fda.gov/downloads/ICECI/Inspections/IOM/UCM135835.pdf
Morris JC. *Dietitian's Guide to Assessment and Documentation.* Sudbury, MA: Jones & Bartlett Learning; 2011.

Modified barium swallow revealed functional oropharyngeal swallow, but moderate-to-severe esophageal dysphagia with delayed movement of liquids in upper esophagus and reflux into pharynx.

3. Nutrition-Focused Physical Findings.

Appears weak and uncomfortable. Reports sore throat, cough, odyno-phagia, and dysphagia.

4. Client History.

He has a 30 pack per year history of smoking, and drinks 3–4 martinis on weekends.

5. Food/Nutrition-Related History.

Recently has been eating only small amounts of scrambled egg, oatmeal, apple juice, canned peaches, and soup.

Medications

He is currently on intravenous fluids and a full liquid diet as tolerated. Medications include ondanestron, hydromorphone, and lansoprazole.

QUESTIONS

1. What risk factors does this client have for esophageal cancer?
2. What is his ideal body weight, BMI, and percentage of both IBW and UBW? Comment on his recent weight change and nutritional status. Calculate his energy, protein, and fluid needs.
3. List the nutrition-related side effects of the chemotherapeutic agents that he will be receiving. What are the possible nutrition-related side effects of radiation treatment?
4. Do you think he will be able to take sufficient nutrition by mouth during his chemotherapy and radiation? Why or why not?
5. What specific dietary interventions could be used to attempt oral nutrition support before the esophagectomy and surgical j-tube are performed?
6. Assuming gastric access can be obtained preoperatively, suggest an enteral feeding regimen that would provide sufficient calories, protein, and fluid for him using an intermittent feeding schedule given over 30–45 minutes 4–6 times daily. Include the formula you choose, the starting volume, how you would advance the feeding, and what your goal volume for formula and flushes

would be. Show your work. Refer to Appendix B for enteral formula information.

7. How would your feeding recommendations change if the formula were given via a jejunostomy tube? Specify the starting rate, how you would advance the feeding, and what your goal rate for formula and flushes would be. Show your work.

8. After he has the partial esophagectomy with reanastamosis and is able to eat by mouth, what type of diet should be recommended?

9. Write a PES statement based on his initial presentation.

10. Write a note that summarizes your assessment in either SOAP or ADIME format.

REFERENCES AND SUGGESTED READINGS

1. Herbella FAM, Harris JE. Esophageal cancer (updated March 8, 2011). Accessed April 21, 2011, from http://emedicine.medscape.com/article/ 277930-overview

2. Loren D, Hashemi N, DiMarino A, Cohen S. Presentation and prognosis of esophageal adenocarcinoma in patients below age 50. *Dig Dis Sci.* 2009; 54: 1708–1712.

3. Bower M, Jones W, Vessels B, Scoggins C, Martin R. Role of esophageal stents in the nutrition support of patients with esophageal malignancy. *Nutr Clin Pract.* 2010; 25:244–249.

4. Bower M, Martin R. Nutritional management during neoadjuvant therapy for esophageal cancer. *J Surg Oncol.* 2009; 100:82–87.

5. Kight C. Nutrition considerations in esophagectomy patients. *Nutr Clin Pract.* 2008; 23:521–528.

6. Joseph M, Meyers MO. Laparoscopic-assisted percutaneous gastrostomy tube placement in the initial management of resectable esophageal and gastroesophageal junction carcinoma. *J Am Coll Surg.* 2010; 211(4):e21–e24.

7. Hurst JD, Gallagher AL. Energy, macronutrient, micronutrient, and fluid requirements. In: Elliot L, Molseed LL, McCallum PD, eds. *The Clinical Guide to Oncology Nutrition*, 2nd ed. Chicago, IL: The American Dietetic Association; 2006; 54–71.

8. Bankhead R, Boullata J, Brantley S, et al. Enteral nutrition practice recommendations. *JPEN J Parenter Enter Nutr.* 2009; 33(2):122–167.

9. American Dietetic Association (ADA). *International Dietetics & Nutrition Terminology (IDNT) Reference Manual: Standardized Language for the Nutrition Care Process*, 3rd edition. Chicago, IL: ADA; 2010.

HIV/AIDS with Wasting

LEARNING OBJECTIVES

Upon completing this case study, readers will be able to:

1. Assess the nutritional status of a patient with HIV/AIDS.
2. Discuss what factors determine an AIDS-defining illness.
3. Determine the side effects of highly active antiretroviral therapy (HAART) as well as the body changes that often accompany HIV/AIDS.
4. Identify the goals of diet therapy and outcomes for monitoring and evaluation of a patient with HIV/AIDS.

CASE DESCRIPTION/BACKGROUND

Poor nutritional status in human immunodeficiency virus (HIV) patients is known to adversely affect the immune system. There are a myriad of nutritional issues associated with the HIV/acquired immunodeficiency syndrome (AIDS) patient such as micronutrient deficiencies, metabolic syndrome, lipodystrophy, obesity, muscle wasting, nausea, and diarrhea. Unintentional weight loss for HIV-positive patients is still associated with high morbidity and mortality (1,2). A visit with a registered dietitian is crucial to decrease the risk of malnutrition in HIV infected patients (3).

The client is a 50-year-old Caucasian man with a history of renal cancer (currently in remission), diverticulosis, hyperlipidemia, sleep apnea, and pancytopenia. His past surgical history includes right partial nephrectomy and clavicle repair. He recently tested positive for HIV during a hospital admission for persistent fever, diarrhea, and abdominal pain. He was also diagnosed with an opportunistic infection; mycobacterium avium complex (MAC) while in the hospital and later was diagnosed with Karposi's sarcoma.

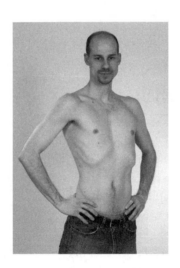

NUTRITIONAL ASSESSMENT DATA

1. Anthropometric Measurements.

Height: 70″
Weight: 184 lbs
Usual weight: 254 lbs
Weight change: 70 lb weight loss in past year

2. Biochemical Data.

Parameter	Value	Normal Values* (may vary by age, sex, and lab)
Viral load	1,287,947 copies/mL	< 48 copies/mL
CD4 lymphocyte	5 cells/mm^3	500–1600 cells/mm^3
Hemoglobin	10.1 g/dL	Male 14–18 g/dL
White blood cells	2900/μL	5000–10,000/μL
Sodium	141 mEq/L	135–147 mEq/L
Potassium	4.5 mEq/L	3.5–5.0 mEq/L
Chloride	107 mEq/L	98–106 mEq/L
BUN	19 mg/dL	8–23 mg/dL
Creatinine	0.8 mg/dL	0.7–1.5 mg/dL
Glucose	94 mg/dL	70–110 mg/dL
Calcium	8.3 mg/dL	8.5–10.8 mg/dL
Albumin	3.5 g/dL	3.5–5.5 g/dL
Cholesterol	151 mg/dL	< 200 mg/dL
LDL	78 mg/dL	< 100 mg/dL
HDL	37 mg/dL	> 40 mg/dL (men)
Triglycerides	151 mg/dL	< 150 mg/dL

*Data from U.S. Food and Drug Administration (FDA). *Investigations Operations Manual.* Silver Spring, MD: US FDA; 2001. Accessed April 21, 2011, from http://www.fda.gov/downloads/ICECI/Inspections/IOM/UCM135835.pdf
Morris JC. *Dietitian's Guide to Assessment and Documentation.* Sudbury, MA: Jones & Bartlett Learning; 2011.

3. Nutrition-Focused Physical Findings.

Patient is alert and oriented. He appears at an appropriate weight for height, although he does appear to have some facial wasting with lesions on his face. His oral health is good. He is complaining of diarrhea and poor energy level, which has been ongoing for the past several months. Patient refused bioelectrical impedance analysis.

4. Client History.

Social Hx

He is currently on disability for a brachial plexis injury, which has been causing some arm pain. He has a history of alcohol abuse and tobacco use. He is currently being followed at an outpatient HIV center.

5. Food/Nutrition-Related History.

The patient reports that he usually has two meals per day. His wife usually prepares most meals. Generally skips lunch secondary to exhaustion. The following is a 24-hour recall.

Usual Diet

Breakfast

Breakfast-type sandwich from a donut shop (ham, egg, and cheese on bagel)
Small coffee with cream and sugar

Snack

Snacks throughout the day
1 apple
2 mini Snickers bars
16 oz water

Dinner

5 oz baked chicken
1 cup rice
1 cup broccoli
1 tbs butter

Medications

Fosamprenavir, ritonavir, Truvada (emtricitabine and tenofovir), simvastatin, pravastatin, bupropion, ranitidine, co-trimoxazole, clarithromycin, azithromycin

Supplements

Vitamin B$_{12}$, 1000 mg (prescribed)

QUESTIONS

1. Calculate his BMI, % IBW, and percentage of weight loss. Define AIDS-related wasting syndrome. Does this patient meet the definition for wasting?
2. What is bioelectrical impedance analysis (BIA)? How would this test have helped to better assess this patient's weight loss? What body changes can occur with HIV infection? Is this patient at risk?
3. Calculate patient's caloric and protein needs. Show your work. What factors would affect this patient's estimated nutritional needs?
4. How is AIDS defined? Does this patient fit the definition? Why?
5. Comment on the adequacy of this patient's current diet. Is he meeting his estimated nutritional needs with current diet? What factors are affecting his food intake?
6. What micronutrients is this patient at risk for becoming deficient in secondary to his disease state? Would you recommend any vitamin or mineral supplements for this patient?
7. Discuss the side effects of this patient's antiretroviral therapy. What nutritional considerations are there with his medications?
8. Considering this patient's CD4 count, he is at increased risk for infection. What education would you provide this patient to decrease his risk of food borne illness?
9. The patient tells you that he has been thinking about starting garlic supplements because he has heard that garlic has many health benefits, and with his history of hyperlipidemia, he thought the garlic might help. What do you tell him about herbal supplements in general, and specifically about garlic?
10. What are his major goals for nutrition therapy? Write a PES statement. How would you monitor the effectiveness of your interventions?

REFERENCES AND SUGGESTED READINGS

1. Colecraft E. HIV/AIDS: nutritional implications and impact on human development. *Proc Nutr Soc.* 2008; 67:109–113.
2. Grinspoon S, Mulligan K. Weight loss and wasting in patients infected with human immunodeficiency virus. Department of Health and Human Services

Working Group on the Prevention and Treatment of Wasting and Weight Loss. 2003; 36(Suppl 2):S69–S78.

3. Position of the American Dietetic Association: nutrition intervention and human immunodeficiency virus infection. *J Am Diet Assoc.* 2010; 110: 1105–1119.

4. Batterham M, Garsia R, Greenop P. Measurement of body composition in people with HIV/AIDS: a comparison of bioelectrical impedance and skinfold antropometry with dual energy x-ray absorptiometry. *J Am Diet Assoc.* 1999; 99(9):1109–1111.

5. Hendricks K, Dong K, Gerrior J, et al. *Nutrition Management of HIV and AIDS.* Chicago, IL: American Dietetic Association; 2009.

6. 1993 revised classification system for HIV infection and expanded surveillance case definition for AIDS among adolescents and adults. *MMWR Recommendations and Reports.* 1993; 41(RR-17):961–962. Accessed April 21, 2011, from http://www.cdc.gov/mmwr/preview/mmwrhtml/00018179.htm

7. Lee LS, Andrade AS, Flexner C. Interactions between natural health products and antiretroviral drugs: pharmacokinetic and pharmacodynamic effects. *Clin Infect Dis.* 2006; 43:1052–1059.

8. Izzo AA, Ernst E. Interactions between herbal medicines and prescribed drugs: an updated systematic review. *Drugs.* 2009; 69(13):1777–1798.

9. Robertson SM, Penzak SR, Pau A. Drug interactions in the management of HIV infection: an update. *Expert Opin Pharmacother.* 2007; (17):2947–2963.

10. American Dietetic Association (ADA). *International Dietetics & Nutrition Terminology (IDNT) Reference Manual: Standardized Language for the Nutrition Care Process*, 3rd ed. Chicago, IL: ADA; 2010.

Gastrointestinal and Nutrition Support

Exacerbation of Crohn's Disease

LEARNING OBJECTIVES

Upon completing this case study, readers will be able to:

1. Identify normal gastrointestinal anatomy and sites of nutrient absorption.
2. Assess the nutritional status of a patient with Crohn's disease.
3. Identify mechanisms for malnutrition in Crohn's disease.
4. Recognize foods that could exacerbate or ameliorate symptoms of diarrhea.
5. Discuss appropriate use of specialized nutrition support in Crohn's disease.

CASE DESCRIPTION/BACKGROUND

Crohn's disease (CD) is a form of inflammatory bowel disease (IBD) that can involve any part of the gastrointestinal tract from the mouth to the perianal area, unlike ulcerative colitis (UC), which only affects the colon (1). Whereas UC causes inflammation limited to the superficial lining of the colon, CD causes inflammation involving the full thickness of the wall of the involved part of the gastrointestinal (GI) tract. CD most commonly affects the end of the small intestine (ileum) and colon (often on the right side) (2). Because CD causes transmural inflammation of the GI tract, the disease can be complicated by inflammatory and fibrous strictures and fistula formation (abnormal communications between organs; e.g., enteroenteral, enterocolonic, enterovesicle, enterocutaneous, and rectovaginal fistulae) (3).

The major symptoms of Crohn's disease include abdominal pain, most commonly in the right lower abdomen, and diarrhea. Rectal bleeding, weight loss, nausea, and vomiting may occur frequently as well (1). Diarrhea may be caused by several factors. Inflammation of the small and large intestines may impair nutrient and fluid absorption. Because bile salts excreted by the liver are reabsorbed by the ileum, ileal disease may prevent bile salt absorption, causing the bile salts to initiate secretion of fluid in the colon. Strictures of the ileum may cause stagnation of GI contents, leading to bacterial overgrowth, another cause of diarrhea in Crohn's patients. If patients have had extensive small bowel surgical resections they may have a so-called "short gut syndrome" with inability to absorb nutrients and fluid (3).

Management of CD involves both drugs and nutritional therapy. In severe cases, surgery may be required. Therapeutic strategy depends on the severity and extent of the disease. Drug therapy can range from a 5-aminosylicylic acid (5-ASA) drug like sulfasalazine or mesalamine alone in mild cases, to steroid therapy, immunosuppressive agents like azathioprine or 6-mercaptopurine, or even biologic agents (monoclonal antibodies to TNFα) in severe cases (1,4). Malnutrition is common in Crohn's disease as a result of inadequate intake, altered absorption, nutrient losses, and in some cases, drug–nutrient interactions (2,5,6). Nutritional therapy may simply involve a regular well-balanced diet in patients with mild disease. Alternatively, a more restrictive low fat, low lactose, and low residue diet may be needed in patients with more extensive disease and those who have had part of their intestine removed. Some patients with severe disease may require enteral supplements (polymeric or even chemically defined), or total parenteral nutrition (TPN) with nothing to eat by mouth (NPO). The use of enteral feedings to both suppress Crohn's disease activity and supplement nutrition is more common in the pediatric population, where maintenance of growth is crucial (7,8).

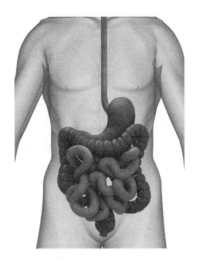

The patient is a 34-year-old woman with a 10-year history of Crohn's ileocolitis. She presents with diarrhea, abdominal pain, and weight loss for the past three weeks, which has not responded to treatment with mesalamine and budesonide. She also has a past medical history of nephrolithiasis. She is a single mother who works full-time as an operating room assistant and has three school-age children.

NUTRITIONAL ASSESSMENT DATA

1. Anthropometric Measurements.

Height: 5'4"
Weight: 140 lbs
Usual weight: 150 lbs
Weight change: Lost 10 lbs in past 3 weeks.

2. Biochemical Data and Test Results.

a. Labs

Parameter	Value	Normal Range* (may vary by age, sex, and lab)
Sodium	145 mEq/L	135–147 mEq/L
Potassium	3.6 mEq/L	3.5–5.0 mEq/L

(continues)

(Continued)

Parameter	Value	Normal Range* (may vary by age, sex, and lab)	
Chloride	110 mEq/L	98–106 mEq/L	H
Carbon dioxide	22 mEq/L	21–30 mEq/L	
BUN	32 mg/dL	8–23 mg/dL	H
Creatinine	1.3 mg/dL	0.7–1.5 mg/dL	
Glucose	140 mg/dL	70–110 mg/dL	H
Hemoglobin	10.8 g/dL	14–18 g/dL (men) 12–16 g/dL (women)	L
Hematocrit	34%	38–54% (men) 36–47% (women)	L
MCV	81 μm³	80.0–94 μm³	
Albumin	3.0 g/dL	3.5–5.5 g/dL	L
C-reactive protein	6 mg/L	0.08–3.10 mg/L	H
Folate	3 μg/L	2–10 μg/L	
Vitamin B₁₂	162 ng/L	200–1000 ng/L	L
Iron	20 μg/L	50–175 μg/dL	L
Ferritin	6 ng/mL	12–150 ng/mL (women) 15–200 ng/mL (men)	L

*Adapted from U. S. Food and Drug Administration. *Investigations Operations Manual.* Silver Spring, MD: US FDA; 2001. Accessed April 21, 2011, from http://www.fda.gov/downloads/ICECI/Inspections/IOM/UCM135835.pdf

Morris JC. *Dietitian's Guide to Assessment and Documentation.* Sudbury, MA: Jones & Bartlett Learning; 2011.

Kratz A, Ferraro M, Sluss PM, Lewandrowski KB. Laboratory reference values. *N Engl J Med.* 2004; 351(15):1548–1563.

b. Pertinent test results

CT scan of abdomen and pelvis revealed thickening of terminal ileum and cecum and inflammatory changes in the mesenteric fat along the right colon. Nephrolithiasis noted in kidney. No obstruction of the small bowel was noted.

3. Nutrition-Focused Physical Findings.

Abdominal exam revealed mild right lower quadrant (RLQ) tenderness with no guarding or rebound. Temperature was 100.8°F. Pulse 112 bpm. Blood pressure 95/65 mm Hg. Respirations 20 breaths per minute.

4. Client History.

Social Hx

She smokes ½ pack per day. Drinks alcohol rarely.

Family Hx

Non-contibutory.

5. Food/Nutrition-Related History.

Usual diet prior to present illness: The patient generally skips breakfast. She eats lunch in the cafeteria at work, where she often chooses salad bar with iceberg lettuce, chicken salad, macaroni salad, cheese, croutons, and creamy dressing. She drinks a large serving of fruit drink. When she gets home from work, she gets busy with her children's activities and homework, and often relies on fast food. Sometimes she heats up frozen chicken nuggets and French fries or macaroni and cheese for dinner, along with some canned fruit in syrup. She drinks chocolate milk with dinner. At night she has a bowl of ice cream with her kids before going to bed.

Over the past three weeks, she has been taking mostly liquids due to her pain and diarrhea. She primarily drinks fruit punch and tea.

Medications

Mesalamine 4.8 g/day, budesonide 9 mg daily. Started on IV methylprednisone 20 mg every twelve hours.

Supplements

None.

QUESTIONS

1. Draw a picture of the GI tract and specify where specific macro- and micronutrients are digested and absorbed.
2. What factors led to inadequate intake in this patient? What percentage of her UBW has she lost? What are some other factors that might lead to poor intake in individuals with CD?
3. What specific nutrients might she have difficulty absorbing due to her ileal disease? Which nutrients might be at risk due to drug–nutrient interactions?

4. What nutrients is she likely to be losing in the diarrhea?
5. What is C-reactive protein and how might it be used in this type of patient? Which of her biochemical lab values indicate that she is anemic and why?
6. Is her nephrolithiasis history related to her CD, and if so, why? Are there nutritional measures that could help to decrease her risk for further problems with kidney stones?
7. What type of oral diet would you recommend for her in the short term?
8. Under what circumstances would you consider enteral or parenteral nutrition for an individual with Crohn's?
9. Identify an appropriate nutrition diagnosis and write a PES statement based on the available nutritional assessment data.
10. What are your goals for this patient, and how would you monitor the effectiveness of your treatment?

REFERENCES AND SUGGESTED READINGS

1. Baumgart DC, Sandborn WJ. Inflammatory bowel disease: clinical aspects and established and evolving therapies. *Lancet.* 2007; 369:1641–1657.
2. Eiden KA. Nutritional considerations in inflammatory bowel disease. *Pract Gastroenterol.* 2003; XXVII(5):33–54.
3. Lichtenstein GR, Hanauer SB, Sandborn WJ. Practice Parameters Committee of American College of Gastroenterology. Management of Crohn's disease in adults. *Am J Gastroenterol.* 2009; 104(2):465–483.
4. Cummings JR, Keshav S, Travis SP. Medical management of Crohn's disease. *BMJ.* 2008; 336(7652):1062–1066.
5. Lucendo AJ, Rezende LC. Importance of nutrition in inflammatory bowel disease. *World J Gastroenterol.* 2009; 15(17):2081–2088.
6. Hartman C, Eliakim R, Shamir R. Nutritional status and nutritional therapy in inflammatory bowel diseases. *World J Gastroenterol* 2009; 15(21): 2570–2578.
7. Rajendran N, Kumar D. Role of diet in the management of inflammatory bowel disease. *World J Gastroenterol.* 2010; 16(12):1442–1448.
8. Moorthy D, Cappellano K, Rosenberg IH. Nutriton and Crohn's disease: an update of print and web-based guidance. *Nutr Rev.* 2008; 66(7):387–397.
9. Insel P, Turner RE, Ross D. *Nutrition,* 3rd ed. Sudbury, MA: Jones and Bartlett Publisher; 2007.
10. United States Department of Agriculture (USDA). MyPyramid Tracker (2011). Accessed April 21, 2011, from http://www.mypyramidtracker.gov/

11. Vermeire S, Van Assche G, Rutgeerts P. C-Reactive Protein as a Marker for Inflammatory Bowel Disease. *Inflamm Bowel Dis.* 2004;10:661–665.

12. Dasher K, Worthington M. Iron: not too much and not too little. *Pract Gastroenterol.* 2009; February:16–26.

13. Kane S. Urogenital Complications of Crohn's dsease. *Am J Gastroenterol.* 2006; 101(12 Suppl):S640–S643.

14. Zachos M, Tondeur M, Griffiths AM. Enteral nutritional therapy for induction of remission in Crohn's disease. *Cochrane Database Syst Rev.* 2007; 1: CD000542. DOI: 10.1002/14651858.CD000542.pub2.

15. American Dietetic Association (ADA). *International Dietetics & Nutrition Terminology (IDNT) Reference Manual: Standardized Language for the Nutrition Care Process*, 3rd ed. Chicago, IL: American Dietetic Association; 2010.

Nutrition Support of the Critically Ill Trauma Patient

LEARNING OBJECTIVES

Upon completion of this case study, readers will be able to:

1. Calculate calorie and protein requirements for trauma patients.
2. Identify situations where an immune-enhancing enteral formula may be appropriate.
3. Recognize factors that affect body weight in the critical care setting.
4. Transition a patient from parenteral to enteral nutrition support.
5. Recognize appropriate methods for monitoring the adequacy of the nutrition support regimen.

CASE DESCRIPTION/BACKGROUND

Trauma is the leading cause of death in Americans between the ages of 1–38 years, resulting in approximately 100,000 deaths per year (1). Traumatic injuries include minor abrasions, contusions, and severe injuries that warrant emergent surgical procedures and extended stays in the intensive care unit (ICU). *Trauma* is typically characterized as blunt versus penetrating trauma, with burns considered separately. Motor vehicle collisions and falls are the most frequent causes of blunt trauma injuries. Penetrating trauma is the result of a stab wound or gunshot wound. Stab wounds generally cause injury only to the immediate penetrating area. In comparison, gunshot wounds may result in injuries to distant tissues.

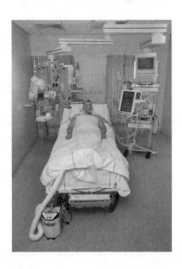

The patient is a 25-year-old man who was admitted to the emergency department secondary to gunshot wounds to the left flank, right buttock, and right thigh. He was taken to the operating room for an exploratory laparotomy, extensive lysis of adhesions, small bowel resection, repair of the third portion of the duodenum, repair of the duodenal wall gunshot wound defect, and feeding jejunostomy. A nasogastric tube was placed for gastric decompression. It was determined by the treatment team that total parenteral nutrition (TPN) would be initiated rather than enteral feedings due to the patient's hemodynamic instability. The RD is consulted for an initial nutritional assessment.

The patient was intubated and sedated during the initial nutrition evaluation. Pertinent weight and diet history information was obtained from the patient's family. His past medical history included a right hemicolectomy, colostomy, and colostomy reversal as a result of a previous gunshot wound. His weight was stable prior to admission, and he did not have any difficulties eating.

On hospital day 10, his abdomen was persistently distended and tympanic. He had an increasing fever and elevated white blood cell count.

He was taken back to the operating room for abdominal re-exploration and underwent an exploratory laparotomy, incision and drainage of a right upper quadrant abscess, duodenum repair, and revision of the feeding jejunostomy secondary to breakdown of the prior duodenal repair.

NUTRITION ASSESSMENT DATA

1. Anthropometric Measurements.

Height: 182.9 cm (72″)
Weight: 96.8 kg (213 lbs)
Usual body weight: 86 kg (189 lbs)

2. Biochemical Data on Admission.

Parameter	Value	Normal Range* (may vary by age, sex, and lab)
Sodium	139 mEq/L	135–147 mEq/L
Potassium	3.9 mEq/L	3.5–5.0 mEq/L
Chloride	111 mEq/L	98–106 mEq/L
Carbon dioxide	25 mEq/L	21–30 mEq/L
BUN	20 mg/dL	8–23 mg/dL
Creatinine	0.8 mg/dL	0.7–1.5 mg/dL
Glucose	115 mg/d	70–110 mg/dL
Hemoglobin	9.5 g/dL	14–18 g/dL (men)
Hematocrit	29.0%	38%–54%
Phosphorus	4.0 mg/dL	3.0–4.5 mg/dL
Albumin	2.2 g/dL	3.5–5.5 g/dL
Prealbumin	9.8 mg/dL	16–40 mg/dL
Alkaline phosphatase	66 U/L	30–120 U/L
Aspartate aminotransferase	24 U/L	0–35 U/L
Alanine transaminase	30 U/L	0–35 U/L
Triglyceride	130 mg/dL	< 150 mg/dL

*Data from U. S. Food and Drug Administration (FDA). *Investigations Operations Manual.* Silver Spring, MD: US FDA; 2001. Accessed April 21, 2011, from http://www.fda.gov/downloads/ICECI/Inspections/IOM/UCM135835.pdf

Morris JC. *Dietitian's Guide to Assessment and Documentation.* Sudbury, MA: Jones & Bartlett Learning, 2011.

Kratz A, Ferraro M, Sluss PM, Lewandrowski KB. Laboratory Reference Values. *N Engl J Med.* 2004; 351:1548–1563.

3. Nutrition-Focused Physical Findings.

He appeared edematous without any obvious signs of nutrient deficiencies.

4. Patient History.

Social History

The patient lived with his mother and two younger siblings.

5. Food/Nutrition-Related History.

The patient's mother reported that the patient did not follow any special diet and had no food allergies or intolerances. She was unable to provide any specifics regarding usual dietary patterns.

QUESTIONS

1. What are the patients' initial calorie and protein requirements? How would you meet his needs with TPN? How many grams of amino acid, dextrose, and lipid would you suggest?
2. Why is the patient's UBW used to determine initial calorie and protein needs as compared to the actual weight after admission to the ICU?
3. Explain why the initial albumin and prealbumin levels are depressed in a patient well-nourished prior to admission without any underlying chronic diseases that would affect nutritional status.
4. Five days following the patient's return to the operating room (hospital day #15), it was decided to initiate enteral nutrition support. Is an immune-enhancing enteral formula indicated at this time? Why or why not?
5. When it was deemed appropriate to initiate enteral nutrition, it was also noted that the patient's prealbumin level had declined to 8.0 mg/dL from 9.8 mg/dL the previous week. The TPN was providing 2.0 g/protein/kg/day. Should the protein provision be increased in the goal enteral nutrition prescription? What test could be utilized to determine if protein provision was sufficient?
6. How do a trauma patient's energy and protein needs change over time? Would a single measure of energy expenditure via indirect calorimetry be beneficial in determining the adequacy of the patient's nutrition support regimen?

7. Should enteral nutrition support initially be provided as continuous, intermittent, or bolus feedings? Suggest a goal feeding (formula and goal rate) and describe how you would progress to the final feeding. How many kilocalories and grams of protein will be provided? Show your work. At what point should the TPN be discontinued?

8. The patient was receiving continuous jejunal tube feedings at a rate of 50 mL/h and a gastric residual volume was 100 mL/h. Is this an indication of intolerance to enteral nutrition?

9. Identify an appropriate nutrition diagnosis for your original evaluation, and write a PES statement based on the available nutritional assessment data.

10. What nutrition-related outcomes would you like to see for this patient?

REFERENCES AND SUGGESTED READINGS

1. Cresci GA, Gottschlich MM, Mayes T, Mueller C. Trauma, surgery, and burns. In: Gottschlich MM, DeLegge MH, Mattox T, Mueller C, Worthington P, eds. *The A.S.P.E.N. Nutrition Support Core Curriculum: A Case-Based Approach- The Adult Patient.* Silver Spring, MD: American Society for Parenteral and Enteral Nutrition; 2007: 455–476.

2. Jacobs D, Jacobs DO, Kudsk K, et al, for the EAST Practice Management Guidelines Workgroup. Practice management guidelines for nutrition support of the trauma patient. *J Trauma.* 2004; 57:660–679.

3. McClave SA, Martindale RG, Vanek VW, et al. Guidelines for the provision and assessment of nutrition support therapy in the adult critically ill patient: Society of Critical Care Medicine (SCCM) and American Society for Parenteral and Enteral Nutrition (A.S.P.E.N.). *JPEN J Parenter Enteral Nutr.* 2009; 33(3):277–316.

4. Kozar RA, McQuiggan MM, Moore FA. Nutrition support of trauma patients. In: Shikora SA, Martindale RG, Schwaitzberg SD, eds. *Nutritional Considerations in the Intensive Care Unit.* Dubuque, IA: Kendall/Hunt; 2002: 229–244.

5. Kozar RA, McQuiggan MM, Moore FA. Trauma. In: Cresci G, ed. *Nutrition Support for the Critically Ill Patient.* Boca Raton, FL: CRC Press, Taylor & Francis Group; 2005: 421–434.

6. Frankenfield D. Energy expenditure and protein requirements after traumatic injury. *Nutr Clin Pract.* 2006; 21:430–437.

7. Winkler MF. Nutrition assessment and monitoring. In: Cresci G, ed. *Nutrition Support for the Critically Ill Patient.* Boca Raton, FL: CRC Press, Taylor & Francis Group; 2005: 71–81.

8. Martindale RG, Shikora SA, Nishikawa R, Seipler JK. The metabolic response to stress and alterations in nutrient metabolism. In: Shikora SA, Martindale RG, Schwaitzberg SD, eds. *Nutritional Considerations in the Intensive Care Unit.* Dubuque, IA: Kendall/Hunt; 2002: 11–19.

9. Cresci G. Nutrition assessment and monitoring. In: Shikora SA, Martindale RG, Schwaitzberg SD, eds. *Nutrition Considerations in the Intensive Care Unit.* Dubuque, IA: Kendall/Hunt; 2002: 21–30.

10. Lefton J, Halasa Esper D, Kochevar M. Enteral formulations. In: Gottschlich MM, DeLegge MH, Mattox T, Mueller C, Worthington P, eds. *The A.S.P.E.N. Nutrition Support Core-Curriculum: A Case-Based Approach–The Adult Patient.* Silver Spring, MD: The American Society for Parenteral and Enteral Nutrition; 2007: 209–232.

11. Krenitsky, J. Immunonutrition—fact, fancy or folly? *Pract Gastroenterol.* 2006; May:47–68.

12. Wooley JA, Frankenfield D. Energy. In: Gottschlich MM, DeLegge MH, Mattox T, Mueller C, Worthington P, eds. *The A.S.P.E.N Nutrition Support Core Curriculum: A Case-Based Approach–The Adult Patient.* Silver Spring, MD: The American Society for Parenteral and Enteral Nutrition; 2007: 19–32.

13. Parrish C, Krenitsky J, Kusenda C. Enteral feeding challenges. In: Cresci G, ed. *Nutrition Support for the Critically Ill Patient.* Boca Raton, FL: CRC Press, Taylor & Francis Group; 2005: 321–340.

14. Bankhead R, Boullata J, Brantley S, et al. Enteral nutrition practice recommendations. *JPEN J Parenter Enter Nutr.* 2009; 33(2):122–167.

15. Marion M, McGinnis C. Overview of parenteral nutrition. In: Gottschlich MM, DeLegge MH, Mattox T, Mueller C, Worthington P, eds. *The A.S.P.E.N Nutrition Support Core-Curriculum: A Case-Based Approach- The Adult Patient.* Silver Spring, MD: The American Society for Parenteral and Enteral Nutrition; 2007: 187–208.

16. American Dietetic Association (ADA). *International Dietetics & Nutrition Terminology (IDNT) Reference Manual: Standardized Language for the Nutrition Care Process,* 3rd ed. Chicago, IL: American Dietetic Association; 2010.

Nutrition Support for Burns

LEARNING OBJECTIVES

Upon completion of this case study, readers will be able to:

1. Apply nutrition assessment skills to a complex patient.
2. Calculate energy and protein requirements for a burn patient.
3. Discuss the use of indirect calorimetry to determine energy needs.
4. Formulate a nutrition support plan to meet nutritional needs of a burn patient.
5. Evaluate the nutrition plan of care while monitoring a burn patient.

CASE DESCRIPTION/BACKGROUND

Burn injury is one of the most traumatic conditions an individual can experience. After a 1- to 3-day "ebb" phase marked by a decreased metabolic rate, a hypermetabolic "flow" phase follows and can last up to a year post-injury (1). Medical nutrition therapy is a major component in the treatment of thermally injured patients. Nutrition support is essential to replace lost nutrients, maintain immunity, and promote healing (1–4). Determining calorie and protein requirements is an important part of the nutrition assessment. Indirect calorimetry is the ideal method to establish energy needs but if unavailable many predictive equations have been developed. The Harris Benedict, Curreri, and Ireton-Jones formula are commonly used. A recent review of burn equations recommends the methods of Xie and Zawacki (5). Protein needs are high, from 1.5–2 g/kg or up to 20%–25% of total kcals (2,5), and can be monitored by nitrogen balance studies.

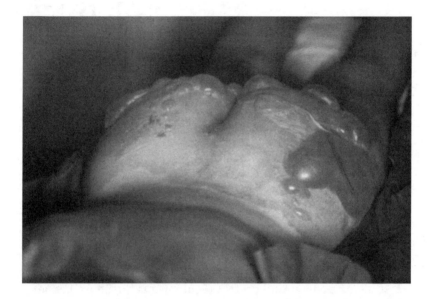

Provision of nutrients can be a challenge. Early enteral nutrition is the norm in most burn units, as it is thought to favorably impact patient outcomes (6–8). A recent multicenter study showed initiation of enteral nutrition within 24 hours of injury prevents ileus, stress ulceration, and the effects of hypermetabolism. Patients who received early enteral nutrition had lower infection rates and shorter ICU length of stays (8). Beta blockers, growth hormone, and anabolic steroids are being used for burn patients to decrease metabolic rate and preserve lean body mass. The use of specialized amino acids and micronutrients are being investigated to improve patient outcomes. Glutamine supplementation has shown significant improvement with infectious complications and length of stay in burn patients. Arginine has a potential role in wound healing, but as yet there are no evidence-based guidelines. Vitamin C is needed for wound healing and has antioxidant properties that are beneficial for burn patients. Selenium may reduce the oxidative stress induced by thermal injury. Supplementation with ornithine alpha-ketoglutarate, Vitamin A, Vitamin D, zinc, and copper may be useful but require further investigation (5). The goals of medical nutrition therapy are fivefold: to lower hypermetabolism, promote healing, reduce infection and oxidative stress, and decrease length of stay (7,8).

The patient is a 47-year-old woman with multiple sclerosis who is confined to a wheelchair. She sustained second- and third-degree burns when her clothing ignited while cooking. She was admitted to a Burn Unit. Initial evaluation determined burns of neck, chest, bilateral upper extremities and anterior thighs with a total burn surface area (TBSA) of 43%. She required escharotomies of chest and left arm. Fluid resuscitation was started at 675 mL/h. Initially, she was able to breathe on her own and did not require mechanical ventilation or enternal feedings. The registered dietitian was consulted for a nutrition assessment.

NUTRITIONAL ASSESSMENT DATA

1. Anthropometric Measurements.

Height: 167.6 cm (5′6″)
Weight: 62.9 kg (138.7 lbs)
Usual weight: 62.7 kg according to the patient
Weight change: stable for the last few years

2. Biochemical Data.

	Post-Burn Day (PBD)									
Parameter	**1**	**5**	**8**	**11**	**13**	**15**	**26**	**29**	**32**	**39**
Glucose mg/dL	127	99	97	113	143	158	183	104	102	134
BUN mg/dL	22	10	20	16	16	14	23	23	41	51
Cr mg/dL	1.1	0.5	0.6	0.5	0.5	0.5	0.5	0.4	0.5	0.6
Na mEq/L	136	136	138	145	141	139	144	146	133	138
K mEq/L	5.4	2.7	3.7	4	3.8	3	4	4	3.7	4
Cl mEq/L	109	115	117	110	109	208	115	117	109	116
CO_2 mEq/L	25	21	19	29	29	27	25	25	21	21

(continues)

(continued)

	Post-Burn Day (PBD)									
Parameter	1	5	8	11	13	15	26	29	32	39
Ca mg/dL	7	6.4	7	7.4	6.9	6.7	7.4	7.1	7.6	7.2
Mg mEq/L	1.4	1.7	1.5	1.6	1.7	1.4	1.8	1.8	1.7	1.6
PO$_4$ mg/dL	6.4	2.1	2.2	1.7	2.6	2.4	2.2	2.4	3.9	2.7
Albumin g/dL	1.7	–	–	1.1	–	1	–	–	–	1
PreAlbumin mg/dL	–	3.5	–	8.4	–	5.3	13.3	–	10.4	21.7
UUN g	–	–	–	–	18	–	–	–	16	–
Weight kg	62.9	80.3	–	75.2	–	77.8	–	–	86.4	–

Test Results

Metabolic cart studies.

PBD	Respiratory Quotient (RQ)	Measured Resting Energy Expenditure (REE) Kcals/day
11	0.71	2538
28	0.79	2438

3. Physical Examination Findings.

The patient was alert and oriented × 3 and appeared well nourished. Second- and third-degree burns were noted on neck, chest, upper extremities, and anterior thighs. Blisters, wound exudate, and blackened skin were noted.

4. Client History.

Social Hx

No smoking, drugs, or alcohol consumption. She does not work and is confined to a wheelchair.

Family Hx

Not applicable.

5. Food/Nutrition History.

She reported a fair appetite with 1-2 meals per day and snacks prior to admission. Her usual intake appeared well balanced. She had no food allergies. She was started on a high protein diet initially.

Medications

No home medications.

Admission Medications

Famotidine, beta carotene, selenium, Vitamin C, Vitamin E, folic acid, multivitamin with minerals, and morphine.

Additional Medications PBD #5

Imipenem, eyrthromycin, ancef, metaclopromide, oxandrin, potassium, and phosphorus.

QUESTIONS

1. Calculate her BMI and body surface area (BSA). Interpret her BMI.
2. Using the Harris Benedict, Curreri, Modified Curreri, Ireton-Jones, Zawacki, and Xie predictive equations found in Appendix A5, what are the patient's estimated energy requirements (EEE)? Compare your results with different equations. Use 1.8–2.0 as stress factors for Harris Benedict.
3. What are her protein requirements?
4. By post burn day (PBD) #5, the patient's condition is deteriorating and she is only taking a few bites of food at each meal. Her respiratory status is also compromised and she will require intubation for ventilator support. How should her nutritional needs be met? Consider alternate types of nutrition support and discuss their risk and benefits (enteral vs. parenteral, gastric vs. post-pyloric feeding).
5. What type of enteral formula would you recommend? Why? What macro- and micronutrients are of particular concern in burn patients? Select a formula, state what the goal would be, and the quantity of macronutrients and fluids provided at goal.

6. The patient had two metabolic cart studies. What is the respiratory quotient? Are the respiratory quotients (RQs) in a physiological range, and why would that matter? What factors can affect the accuracy of metabolic cart studies?

7. How should a measured resting energy expenditure (MREE) be used to calculate energy needs? What factor would be applied to the MREE for a burn patient? What changes should be made to the nutrition regimen that you recommended in question 5 after study PBD #11?

8. The patient had two 24-hour urine collections for UUN. Assuming that tube feeds were being tolerated at goal and burn size is reduced to 20% TBSA, what is the N balance on PBD #13? What changes, if any, are needed to the nutrition regimen? Use the following formula for nitrogen balance (15):

$$N_{IN} = N_{OUT} = UUN + \text{Insensible Loss (4)} + \text{Burn Loss (0.05 gN/kg)}$$

9. On PDB #14, the patient was extubated and had a Speech Language Swallowing Evaluation on PBD #15. She was cleared for a pureed diet with honey thick liquids. What changes should be made to the nutrition regimen?

10. Write a PES statement based on available assessment data on PBD #5. Name specific interventions that would address her nutrition diagnosis, and specify how you would monitor their effectiveness.

REFERENCES AND SUGGESTED READINGS

1. Lee JO, Benjamin D, Herndon DN. Nutrition support strategies for severely burned patients. *Nutr Clin Pract.* 2005; 20:325–330.
2. Prelack K, Dylewski M, Sheridan R. Practice guidelines for nutritional management of burn injury and recovery. *J Burns.* 2007; 33:14–24.
3. Wolf SE. Nutrition and metabolism in burns: state of the science, 2007. *J Burn Care Res.* 2007; 28(4):572–576.
4. Graves C, Saffle J, Cochran A. Actual burn nutrition care practices: an update. *J Burn Care Res.* 2009; 30:77–82.
5. Sullivan J. Nutrition and metabolic support in severe burn injury. *Support Line.* 2010; 32(2):3–13.

6. Saffle J, Arenholz D, Cope N, et al. Practice guidelines for burn care. *J Burn Care Rehab.* 2001; (22):S1–S69.

7. McClave SA, Martindale RG, Vanek VW, et al. Guidelines for the provision and assessment of nutrition support therapy in the adult critically ill patient: Society of Critical Care Medicine (SCCM) and American Society for Parenteral and Enteral Nutrition (A.S.P.E.N.). *JPEN J Parenter Enteral Nutr.* 2009; 33(3):277–316.

8. Mosier M, Pham T, Klein M, et al. Early enteral nutrition in burns: compliance with guidelines and associated outcomes in a multi-center study. *J Burn Care Res.* 2011; 32:104–109.

9. Pesce-Hammond K, Wessel J. Nutrition assessment and decision making. In: Merritt R, ed. *The A.S.P.E.N. Nutrition Support Practice Manual.* Silver Spring, MD; 2005: 3–26.

10. Mosteller RD. Simplified calculation of body surface area. *N Engl J Med.* 1987: 317(17):1098.

11. Ireton-Jones C, Jones JD. Improved equations for predicting energy expenditure in patients: the Ireton-Jones equations. *Nutr Clin Pract.* 2002; 17:29–31.

12. Dickerson R, Gervasio J, Riley M, et al. Accuracy of predictive methods to estimate resting energy expenditure of thermally-injured patients. *JPEN J Parenter Enter Nutr.* 2002; 26:17–29.

13. Curreri PW, Richmond D, Marvin J, Baxter CR. Classic article: dietary requirements of patients with major burns. *Nutr Clin Pract.* 2001; 16: 169–171.

14. McClave SA, Lowen CC, Kleber MJ, McConnell JW, Jung LY, Goldsmith LJ. Clinical use of the respiratory quotient obtained from indirect calorimetry. *JPEN J Parenter Enteral Nutr.* 2003; 27: 21–26.

15. Gottschlich M, Mayes T. Burns. In: Merritt R, ed. *The A.S.P.E.N. Nutrition Support Practice Manual.* Silver Spring, MD: American Society for Parenteral and Enteral Nutrition; 2005: 296–300.

16. American Dietetic Association (ADA). *International Dietetics & Nutrition Terminology (IDNT) Reference Manual: Standardized Language for the Nutrition Care Process*, 3rd ed. Chicago, IL: ADA; 2010.

Tools for Assessment and Monitoring

A1. CLINICAL CONVERSIONS

Measures of Volume

Common Measure	Abbreviation	Equivalency	Metric Measure
1 cup	–	8 oz	240 mL
1 ounce (liquid)	oz		29.57 mL
1 teaspoon	tsp		5 mL
1 tablespoon	tbs	3 tsp	15 mL

Measures of Weight and Length

Common Measure	Equivalency	Metric Measure
1 pound (lb)		0.45 kilogram (kg)
1 inch (")		2.54 centimeters (cm)
3.28 feet (')	1 meter (m)	100 (cm)

Commonly Used Conversions

To Convert	Use
Pounds to kilograms	Divide pounds by 2.2
Inches to centimeters	Multiply inches by 2.54
Centimeters to meters	Divide centimeters by 100

A2. WEIGHT CALCULATIONS

Parameter	Equation
IBW	Hamwi equation (1) • Males 106 lbs for the first 5 feet, + 6 lbs for every inch over 5 feet, ± 10% • Females 100 lbs for first 5 feet, + 5 lbs for every inch over 5 feet, ± 10%
Percent IBW	% IBW = (current weight ÷ IBW) × 100
Percent UBW	% UBW = (current weight ÷ usual weight) × 100
Percent weight loss*	% Weight Loss = (usual weight − current weight) ÷ usual weight

*Note: Weight loss of > 5% in one month or > 10% in 6 months is considered clinically significant (2).
Abbreviations: IBW, ideal body weight; UBW, usual body weight.

A3. BODY MASS INDEX (BMI) CALCULATIONS

Calculation of BMI

To calculate BMI for adults and children, use the following formulas:

Measurement Units	Formula Notes
Kilograms and meters (or centimeters)	weight (kg) / [height (m)]^2 With the metric system, the formula for BMI is weight in kilograms divided by height in meters squared. Because height is commonly measured in centimeters, divide height in centimeters by 100 to obtain height in meters. Example: weight = 68 kg, height = 165 cm (1.65 m) Calculation: $68 \div (1.65)^2 = 24.98$

(Continued)

Measurement Units	Formula Notes
Pounds and inches	weight / [height]^2 × 703 Calculate BMI by dividing weight in pounds (lbs) by height in inches (") squared and multiplying by a conversion factor of 703. Example: weight = 150 lbs, height = 5'5" (65") Calculation: [150 ÷ (65)^2] × 703 = 24.96

Source: Centers for Disease Control and Prevention. Available at: http://www.cdc.gov/healthyweight/assessing/bmi/adult_bmi/index.html

Interpretation of BMI for Adults

Over 20 years of age, BMI is interpreted the same way for both men and women regardless of age.

BMI (kg/m^2)	Weight Status
< 18.5	Underweight
18.5–24.9	Normal
25.0–29.9	Overweight
≥ 30.0	Obese

Source: Centers for Disease Control and Prevention. Available at: http://www.cdc.gov/healthyweight/assessing/bmi/adult_bmi/index.html

Interpretation of BMI for Children and Teens

For children age two and teens through age 19, the interpretation of BMI is sex-specific, and based on percentiles for age. After calculating the BMI, it should be plotted on the sex-specific growth chart and compared to percentiles using the Center for Disease Control and Prevention (CDC)'s BMI for age charts (refer to the appropriate charts at: http://www.cdc.gov/growthcharts/clinical_charts.htm). Weight status for calculated BMI for age can be interpreted using the following table.

Weight Status Category	Percentile Range
Underweight	< 5th percentile
Healthy weight	5th percentile < 85th percentile

(continues)

(Continued)

Weight Status Category	Percentile Range
Overweight	85th < 95th percentile
Obese	≥ 95th percentile

Source: Centers for Disease Control and Prevention. Available at: http://www.cdc.gov/
healthyweight/assessing/bmi/childrens_bmi/about_childrens_bmi.html#How is BMI calculated

A4. ENERGY EQUATIONS

Activity and/or injury factors are commonly applied to equations that estimate basal or resting energy expenditure in order to estimate total energy expenditure. These vary by disease state and tend to be based more on clinical judgment than evidence, particularly when dealing with individual patients. Factors range from 1.0 to 1.2 for sedentary patients with minimal stress, up to 1.5 to 1.6 for those with moderate activity or additional needs for healing, and occasionally up to 2.0 for those with burns, vigorous activity, or malabsorption.

Name Purpose	Equation Notes
Mifflin St. Jeor equation (3) Used for estimating REE in kcal/d	Males: REE = (9.99 × weight) + (6.25 × height) − (4.92 × age) + 5 Females: REE = (9.99 × weight) + (6.25 × height) − (4.92 × age) − 161 *Important:* Use actual weight in kg, height in cm, and age in years. Original authors suggest that 9.99 can be rounded to 10 and 4.92 can be rounded to 5 (3).
Harris Benedict equation (2) Used for estimating BEE in kcal/d	Men: BEE = 66 + (13.7 × weight) + (5.0 × height) − (6.8 × age) Women: 655 + (9.6 × weight) + (1.8 × height) − (4.7 × age) *Important:* Use weight in kg, height in cm, and age in years.

World Health Organization (4)
 	
Used for estimating BMR in kcal/d
	Male < 3 years BMR = 60.9 (weight) − 54
	          3–10 years BMR = 22.7 (weight) + 495
	          10–18 years BMR = 17.5 (weight) + 651
	Female < 3 years BMR = 61.0 (weight) − 51
	          3–10 years BMR = 22.5 (weight) + 499
	          10–18 years BMR = 12.2 (weight) + 746
	Important: Use weight in kg

(Continued)

Catch up growth needs (5) for children with stunted growth	$\text{kcal/kg/d} = \dfrac{\text{RDA for age (kcal/kg)} \times \text{ideal weight for height}}{\text{Actual weight}}$ Grams of protien L/kg/day = $\dfrac{\text{RDA for age (kcal/kg)} \times \text{ideal weight for height}}{\text{Actual weight}}$

Abbreviations: BEE, basal energy expenditure; BMR, basal metabolic rate; RDA, Recommended Daily Allowance; REE, resting energy expenditure.

A5. ENERGY EQUATIONS FOR BURN PATIENTS

Name Purpose	Equation Notes
Curreri equation Used for total caloric goal (6)	Ideal daily caloric intake = $(25 \times \text{weight in kg}) + (40 \times \% \text{ BSAB})$
Modified Curreri equation Used for total caloric goal based on age and sex (7)	Male: Ideal daily caloric intake = $[25 \text{ kcal/kg} \times \text{BMR factor}] + (40 \times \text{BSAB})$ Female: Ideal daily caloric intake = $22 \text{ kcal/kg} \times \text{BMR factor} + (40 \times \text{BSAB})$ BMR factors: 20–40 years old = 1 40–50 years old = 0.95 50–60 years old = 0.90 75–100 years old = 0.80
Zawacki equation Used for EEE (7)	$\text{EEE} = 1440 \text{ calorie/m}^2/\text{d}$
Xie equation Used for EEE (7)	$\text{EEE} = (1000 \text{ calorie/m}^2/\text{d}) + (25 \times \text{BSAB})$
Ireton-Jones equations Used for EEE (8)	Spontaneously breathing: $[629 - 11(A)] + [25 (W) - 609 (O)]$ Ventilator-dependent (2002 equation): $[1784 - 11 (A)] + [5 (W) + 244 (S)] + [239 (T) + 804 (B)]$ A = Age in years B = Diagnosis of burn (present = 1, absent = 0) O = Obesity, BMI >27 kg/m² (present = 1, absent = 0) S = Sex (male = 1, female = 0) T = Diagnosis of trauma (present = 1, absent = 0)

Abbreviations: BSAB, body surface area burned; BMR, basal metabolic rate; BSI, body mass index; d, day; EEE, estimated energy expenditure.

A6. PROTEIN CALCULATIONS

Protein Requirements

Protein needs are increased from the RDA of 0.8 g/kg to 1.0–1.5 g/kg in moderate illness and 1.2–2.0 g/kg in critical illness, possibly higher in burn and multi-trauma patients (2,9).

Nitrogen Balance (2)

Nitrogen balance = Nitrogen "In" (calculated from protein intake)
– Nitrogen "Out" (measured nitrogen losses
+ "fudge factor" for insensible losses)
Nitrogen balance = grams protein/6.25 – grams of urine urea nitrogen + 4

A7. BIOCHEMICAL DATA

Lab Test	Reference Range (may vary by age, sex, and lab)	Partial listing of factors that may affect serum levels
Sodium	135–147 mEq/L	Hyponatremia usually results from fluid overload or sodium losses rather than insufficient dietary intake. It is associated with excessive administration of hypotonic IV fluids, heart failure, severe burns, diarrhea, vomiting, diuretics, SIADH, edema, ascites, diabetic ketoacidosis, and severe nephritis. Hypernatremia can result from dehydration, hyperaldosteronism, Cushing disease, and diabetes insipidus.
Potassium	3.5–5.5 mEq/L	Potassium affects the rate and force of the contraction of heart muscles. Potassium depletion can be commonly caused by gastrointestinal losses and potassium-depleting diuretics. Other factors associated with hypokalemia are hypomagnesemia, metabolic alkalosis, anorexia nervosa, malnutrition, and liver disease with ascites. Hyperkalemia is frequently caused by kidney disease. Cellular damage or hemolysis can release intracellular potassium into the serum and cause hyperkalemia. Hyperkalemia can also result from acidosis, internal hemorrhage, and overuse of potassium supplements.

(Continued)

Lab Test	Reference Range (may vary by age, sex, and lab)	Partial listing of factors that may affect serum levels
Chloride	98–106 mEq/L	Chloride levels tend to change with sodium levels. Serum chloride decreases with severe vomiting, gastric suctioning, diarrhea, severe burns, over-hydration, metabolic alkalosis, and certain diuretics. High chloride levels can occur with metabolic acidosis, dehydration, and excessive IV chloride administration. This is common with normal saline fluid resuscitation producing a hyperchloremic metabolic acidosis, e.g., after fluid resuscitation.
Carbon Dioxide (CO_2)	20–29 mEq/L	Serum CO_2 reflects serum bicarbonate on a routine blood test. Low levels can result from diarrhea, pancreatic fistulae, acidosis, and kidney disease. High levels occur in alkalosis, excessive vomiting, volume contraction (contraction alkalosis), and hyperaldosteronism.
Blood Urea Nitrogen (BUN)	8–23 mg/dL	BUN is an end product of protein metabolism. BUN increases with dehydration, renal dysfunction, high protein intake, protein catabolism, and gastrointestinal hemorrhage. BUN decreases with overhydration, malnutrition, and liver disease.
Creatinine	0.7–1.5 mg/dL	Creatinine is a product of muscle creatine breakdown. It is increased in chronic or acute kidney disease, urinary obstruction, dehydration, and rhabdomyolysis. It may be decreased in malnutrition, muscle wasting, and muscle disorders such as muscular dystrophy.
Glucose	70–110 mg/dL	Serum glucose (blood sugar) levels are regulated by insulin and glucagon. They can be increased by oral intake especially carbohydrates, IV dextrose, steroids, infection, and metabolic stress. Hyperglycemia may occur in diabetes, Cushing syndrome, hyperthyroidism, pancreatitis, pancreatic cancer, and with use of certain medications, notably corticosteroids. Hypoglycemia is associated with excessive insulin administration, liver disease, glycogen storage disease, hypothyroidism, and starvation.

(continues)

(Continued)

Lab Test	Reference Range (may vary by age, sex, and lab)	Partial listing of factors that may affect serum levels
Magnesium	1.8–3.6 mg/dL	Magnesium is a cofactor for many enzymes and also plays a role in the metabolism of other minerals including calcium and potassium. Low levels of magnesium may occur in patients with malnutrition, chronic diarrhea, chronic alcoholism, hepatic cirrhosis, and pregnancy induced hypertension. High levels may occur in kidney disease, Addison's disease, diabetic acidosis, and dehydration.
Phosphorus	3–4.5 mg/dL	Phosphorus is regulated by the kidneys and parathyroid glands. Hyperphosphatemia is common in kidney disease and is also seen in hypoparathyroidism, hypocalcemia, and excessive vitamin D intake. Hypophosphatemia is associated with primary hyperparathyroidism, rickets, osteomalacia, refeeding syndrome, and malnutrition.
Calcium	8.5–10.8 mg/dL	Serum calcium includes both ionized and bound calcium. About half of the serum calcium is bound to albumin, so calcium levels can appear low with hypoalbuminemia. Serum calcium can increase with hyperparathyroidism, cancer, vitamin D toxicity, and immobility. It may be low in hypoparathyroidism, magnesium deficiency, kidney disease, and vitamin D deficiency.
Albumin	3.5–5.5 g/dL	While serum albumin may reflect malnutrition, it can be affected by many factors. Hypoalbuminemia can occur in liver disease due to reduced synthetic capacity, nephrotic syndrome due to urinary losses, fluid overload or edema/ascites due to expanded volume status, and inflammation/infection since it is a negative acute phase protein. Serum albumin may be elevated with dehydration. Because of its 21 day half life, albumin does not reflect acute changes in nutritional status.
Prealbumin (transthyretin)	16–40 mg/dL	Prealbumin may be a more sensitive indicator of nutritional status due to its half-life of about 2 days. It is affected by inflammation and infection, and will drop quickly in response to acute illness. It may be elevated in kidney disease.

(Continued)

Lab Test	Reference Range (may vary by age, sex, and lab)	Partial listing of factors that may affect serum levels
Hemoglobin	12–16 g/dL (women) 14–18 g/dL (men)	Hemoglobin (HGB) is a protein that transports oxygen and carbon dioxide in the blood. Decreased levels of HGB, red blood cells (RBC's), and hematocrit (HCT) indicate anemia. Low HGB levels are also associated with bleeding, overhydration, kidney disease with low erythropoietin production, hemolysis, hemoglobinopathies, cancer, and autoimmune diseases such as systemic lupus erythematosus. Increased levels of hemoglobin are associated with polycythemia, dehydration, chronic obstructive pulmonary disease, heart failure, dehydration, and high altitude.
Hematocrit	36–47% (women) 38–54% (men)	Hematocrit (HCT) is the percent of blood volume that consists of red blood cells (RBC's). HCT can be affected by altitude and hydration status. Low levels indicate anemia and are associated with malnutrition, deficiencies of iron, folate, vitamin B_{12}, and vitamin B_6, and factors related to low hemoglobin (see above). A high HCT is associated with dehydration, high altitude, low oxygen levels, and polycythemia.
Ferritin	12–150 ng/mL (women) 15–200 ng/mL (men)	Ferritin is the principal storage form of iron in the body. Low levels are associated with iron deficiency and bleeding. Inflammatory conditions will raise the ferritin level, and may falsely suggest adequate iron status. Other conditions associated with increased ferritin include hemochromatosis, alcoholic liver disease, and frequent transfusions.
MCV	80–94 μm^3 (cubic micrometers)	The MCV is a measure of the average red blood cell size. It is used to diagnose types of anemia. A low MCV indicates a microcytic anemia, whereas a high MCV indicates a macrocytic anemia. Microcytic anemia is associated with iron deficiency, lead poisoning, thalassemia, and chronic kidney disease. Macrocytic anemia is associated with deficiencies of vitamin B_{12} and folate and some chemotherapies.

(continues)

(Continued)

Lab Test	Reference Range (may vary by age, sex, and lab)	Partial listing of factors that may affect serum levels
MCH	27–32 pg/cell (picograms/cell)	Mean Corpuscular Hemoglobin (MCH) is the amount of hemoglobin per red blood cell. In anemia, a low MCH indicates a hypochromic anemia; a normal MCH a normochromic anemia, and a high MCH a hyperchromic anemia. A hypchromic anemia is associated with iron deficiency.
Glycosylated Hemoglobin (Hb A$_{1C}$)	Nondiabetic: 4.0–6.0% Diabetic: < 6.5–7%	Hb A$_{1C}$ is used to monitor blood sugar control over a 2–3 month period and may also be used as a factor to predict or diagnose diabetes. Higher levels are associated with higher average blood sugars and poor glycemic control. Hemoglobinopathies can result in a falsely low level.
Total Cholesterol	< 200 mg/dL desirable 200–239 mg/dL borderline high > 240 mg/dLHigh	Increased levels of total cholesterol are correlated with the incidence of coronary heart disease. It may be used as a screening tool or in combination with a lipid profile. High levels are associated with a high fat diet, familial hypercholesterolemia, hypothyroidism, nephritic syndrome, pregnancy, and uncontrolled diabetes. Low total cholesterol levels may be a result of malnutrition, malabsorption, hyperthyroidism, liver disease, and sepsis.
LDL Cholesterol	<100 mg/dL Optimal 100–129 mg/dL Near optimal/above optimal 130–159 mg/dL Borderline High	Low density lipoprotein (LDL) cholesterol is also known as "bad cholesterol" and is correlated with coronary heart disease. It is used as a target measure to assess both risk for heart disease and response to therapy. High levels are associated with increased risk of atherosclerotic heart disease and a family history of hyperlipoproteinemia, and may be caused by a diet high in saturated fat and cholesterol. Low levels are associated with malabsorption and malnutrition.

(Continued)

Lab Test	Reference Range (may vary by age, sex, and lab)	Partial listing of factors that may affect serum levels
	160–189 mg/dL High ≥ 190 mg/dL Very High	
HDL Cholesterol	< 40 mg/dL low HDL cholesterol ≥ 60 mg/dL High HDL cholesterol	High density lipoprotein (HDL) is also known as "good cholesterol". Low HDL levels are correlated with increased risk for coronary heart disease and heart attack. Low HDL is associated with genetic factors, smoking, insulin resistance, type 2 diabetes, elevated triglycerides, obesity, and physical inactivity. High levels of HDL reduce risk of coronary heart disease. Physical activity can increase HDL levels. Women tend to have higher HDL than men and may have higher target levels.
Triglycerides	< 150 mg/dL	Increased serum triglycerides often occur along with other conditions that increase risk for heart disease. Serum triglycerides may be increased by excessive alcohol or very high carbohydrate intake, type 2 diabetes, chronic renal failure, pancreatitis, hypothyroidism, nephrotic syndrome, physical inactivity, and overweight and obesity. Low levels are associated with malnutrition, malabsorption, and hyperthyroidism.

Data from: Morris JC, *Dietitian's Guide to Assessment and Documentation.* Sudbury, MA: Jones & Bartlett Learning, 2011; U.S. Food and Drug Administration. *Investigations Operations Manual.* Silver Spring, MD: US FDA; 2001. http://www.fda.gov/downloads/ICECI/Inspections/IOM/UCM135835.pdf. Accessed November 13, 2010; MedlinePlus [Internet]. Bethesda (MD): National Library of Medicine (US); [updated 2011 April 29; cited 2011 May 1]. Available from: http://www.nlm.nih.gov/medlineplus/; American Heart Association. Third Report of the National Cholesterol Education Program (NCEP) Expert Panel on Detection, Evaluation, and Treatment of High Blood Cholesterol in Adults (Adult Treatment Panel III) Final Report. *Circulation* 2002; 106;3143; American Diabetes Association. Diagnosis and Classification of Diabetes Mellitus. *Diabetes Care* 2010; 33: s62–s69.

A8. PHYSICAL INDICATORS OF NUTRITIONAL STATUS

Body Area	Signs of Good Nutrition	Signs of Malnutrition

1. Head to neck
  a. Hair
  b. Face
  c. Eyes
  d. Lips
  e. Tongue
  f. Teeth
  g. Gums
	a. Shiny
	b. Skin smooth
	c. Bright
	d. Smooth
	e. Deep red
	f. Straight; none missing
	g. Firm, pink, smooth, no bleeding
		a. Dull, dry, thin, wire-like, sparse, brittle; scalp rough, flaky
		b. Pale or mottled, dark under eyes, swollen, scaling or flakiness, lumpiness
		c. Dry membranes, redness, fissures at corners, red rimmed, fine blood vessels or scars at cornea
		d. Red, swollen, lesions or fissures
		e. Scarlet or purplish color; raw, swollen, smooth
		f. Cavities, black or gray spots, erupting abnormally, missing
		g. Spongy, bleed easily, inflammation, receded, atrophied

2. Skin	Smooth, moist, uniform color	Dry, flaky, scaling, "gooseflesh," swollen, grayish, bruises due to capillary bleeding under skin, no fat layer under skin
3. Glands	No thyroid enlargement: no lumps at parotid juncture	Front of neck and cheeks become swollen, lumps visible at parotid; goiter visible if advanced hypothyroidism
4. Nails	Pink nail beds, smooth, firm, flexible, uniform shape	Brittle, ridged, pale nail beds, clubbed, spoon shaped
5. Muscle and skeletal system	Good posture, firm, well-developed muscles, good mobility; no malformations of skeleton	Flaccid, wasted muscles, weakness, tenderness, decreased reflexes, difficulty in walking Children: beading ribs, swelling at ends of bones, abnormal protrusion of frontal or parietal areas

(Continued)

Body Area	Signs of Good Nutrition	Signs of Malnutrition

6. Internal systems
  a. Gastrointestinal
  b. Cardiovascular
	a. Flat abdomen, liver not tender to palpate, normal size
	b. Normal pulse rate; normal blood pressure
		a. Distended, enlarged abdomen, ascites, hepatomegaly (enlarged liver)
		Children: "potbelly"
		b. Pulse rate exceeds 100 beats/ min., abnormal rhythm, blood pressure elevated, mental confusion, edema

While physical appearances give us clues to internal problems, they can be misleading. They may not be nutrition related. Physical findings must be coupled with other indications (lab test, anthropometries, etc.) in order to validate them.

A9. FOOD AND DRUG INTERACTIONS

Allergies

Antihistamines are used to relieve or prevent the symptoms of colds, hay fever, and allergies. They limit or block histamine, which is released by the body when we are exposed to substances that cause allergic reactions. Antihistamines are available with and without a prescription (over-the-counter). These products vary in their ability to cause drowsiness and sleepiness.

Antihistamines

Some examples are:
    Over-the-counter:
    brompheniramine / DIMETANE, BROMPHEN
    chlorpheniramine / CHLOR-TRIMETON
    diphenhydramine / BENADRYL
    clemastine / TAVIST
    Prescription:
    fexofenadine / ALLEGRA
    loratadine / CLARITIN (now available over the counter)

cetirizine / ZYRTEC

Interaction

Food: It is best to take prescription antihistamines on an empty stomach to increase their effectiveness.

Alcohol: Some antihistamines may increase drowsiness and slow mental and motor performance. Use caution when operating machinery or driving.

Arthritis and Pain

Analgesic/Antipyretic

They treat mild to moderate pain and fever. An example is: acetaminophen/ TYLENOL.

Interactions

Food: For rapid relief, take on an empty stomach because food may slow the body's absorption of acetaminophen.

Alcohol: Avoid or limit the use of alcohol because chronic alcohol use can increase your risk of liver damage or stomach bleeding. If you consume three or more alcoholic drinks per day talk to your doctor or pharmacist before taking these medications.

Non-Steroidal Anti-Inflammatory Drugs (NSAIDs)

NSAIDs reduce pain, fever, and inflammation.

Some examples are:

aspirin / BAYER, ECOTRIN

ibuprofen / MOTRIN, ADVIL

naproxen / ANAPROX, ALEVE, NAPROSYN

nabumetone / RELAF

celecoxis / CELEBREX

Interaction

Food: Because these medications can irritate the stomach, it is best to take them with food or milk.

Alcohol: Avoid or limit the use of alcohol because chronic alcohol use can increase your risk of liver damage or stomach bleeding. If you consume three or more alcoholic drinks per day, talk to your doctor or pharmacist before taking these medications. Buffered aspirin or enteric coated aspirin may be preferable to regular aspirin to decrease stomach bleeding.

Corticosteroids

They are used to provide relief to inflamed areas of the body. Corticosteroids reduce swelling and itching, and help relieve allergic, rheumatoid, and other conditions.

Some examples are:

methylprednisolone / MEDROL

prednisone / DELTASONE

prednisolone / PEDIAPRED, PRELONE

cortisone acetate / CORTEF

Interaction

Food: Take with food or milk to decrease stomach upset. These medications can lead to negative calcium balance and impaired bone health.

Narcotic Analgesics

Narcotic analgesics are available only with a prescription. They provide relief for moderate to severe pain. Codeine can also be used to suppress cough. Some of these medications can be found in combination with non-narcotic drugs such as acetaminophen, aspirin, or cough syrups. Use caution when taking these medications. Take them only as directed by a doctor or pharmacist because they may be habit-forming and can cause serious side effects when used improperly.

Some examples are:

codeine combined with acetaminophen / TYLENOL #2, #3, and #4

morphine / ROXANOL, MS CONTIN

oxycodone combined with acetaminophen / PERCOCET, ROXICET

meperidine / DEMEROL

hydrocodone with acetaminophen / VICODIN, LORCET

Interaction

Alcohol: Avoid alcohol because it increases the sedative effects of the medications. Use caution when motor skills are required, including operating machinery and driving.

Asthma

Bronchodilators

Bronchodilators are used to treat the symptoms of bronchial asthma, chronic bronchitis, and emphysema. These medicines open air passages to the lungs to relieve wheezing, shortness of breath, and troubled breathing.

Some examples are:

theophylline / SLO-BID, THEO-DUR, THEO-DUR 24, UNIPHYL
albuterol / VENTOLIN, PROVENTIL, COMBIVENT
epinephrine / PRIMATENE MIST
montelukast / SINGULAIR
salmeterol xinefoate / SEREVENT

Interactions

Food: The effect of food on theophylline medications can vary widely. High-fat meals may increase the amount of theophylline in the body while high-protein, low-carb meals, and charcoal-broiled foods may decrease it. It is important to check with your pharmacist about which form you are taking because food can have different effects depending on the dose form (for example, regular release, sustained release, or sprinkles). For example, food has little effect on Theo-Dur and Slo-Bid, but food increases the absorption of Theo-Dur 24 and Uniphyl, which can result in side effects of nausea, vomiting, headache, and irritability. Food can also decrease absorption of products like Theo-Dur Sprinkles for children.

Caffeine: Avoid eating or drinking large amounts of foods and beverages that contain caffeine (for example, chocolate, colas, coffee, tea) because both oral bronchodilators and caffeine stimulate the central nervous system.

Alcohol: Avoid alcohol if you are taking theophylline medications because it can increase the risk of side effects such as nausea, vomiting, headache, and irritability.

Cardiovascular Disorders

There are numerous medications used to treat cardiovascular disorders such as high blood pressure, angina, irregular heartbeat, and high cholesterol. These drugs are often used in combination to enhance their effectiveness. Some classes of drugs can treat several conditions. For example, beta blockers can be used to treat high blood pressure, angina, and irregular heartbeats. Check with your doctor or pharmacist if you have questions on any of your medications. Some of the major cardiovascular drug classes are:

Diuretics

Sometimes called "water pills," diuretics help eliminate water, sodium, and chloride from the body. There are different types of diuretics.

Some examples are:
furosemide / LASIX
triamterene / hydrochlorothiazide / DYAZIDE, MAXZIDE
hydrochlorothiazide / HYDRODIURIL
triamterene / DYRENIUM
bumetamide / BUMEX
metolazone / ZAROXOLYN
Interaction
Food: Diuretics vary in their interactions with food and specific nutrients. Some diuretics cause loss of potassium, calcium, and magnesium. Supplements may be needed. Triamterene, on the other hand, is known as a "potassium-sparing" diuretic. It blocks the kidneys' excretion of potassium, which can cause hyperkalemia (increased potassium). Excess potassium may result in irregular heartbeat and heart palpitations. When taking triamterene; avoid eating large amounts of potassium-rich foods such as bananas, oranges, and green leafy vegetables, or salt substitutes that contain potassium.

Beta Blockers

Beta blockers decrease the nerve impulses to the heart and blood vessels. This decreases the heart rate and the workload of the heart.
Some examples are:
atenolol / TENORMIN
metoprolol / LOPRESSOR
propranolol / INDERAL
nadolol / CORGARD
Interaction
Alcohol: Avoid drinking alcohol with propranolol /INDERAL because the combination lowers blood pressure too much.

Nitrates

Nitrates relax blood vessels and lower the demand for oxygen by the heart.
Some examples are:
isosorbide dinitrate / ISORDIL, SORBITRATE
nitroglycerin / NITRO, NITRO-DUR, TRANSDERM-NITRO, NITROSTAT, NITROLINGUAL SPRAY
Interaction
Alcohol: Avoid alcohol because it may add to the blood vessel-relaxing effect of nitrates and result in dangerously low blood pressure.

Angiotensin Converting Enzyme (ACE) Inhibitors

ACE inhibitors relax blood vessels by preventing angiotensin II, a vaso-constrictor, from being formed.

Some examples are:

captopril / CAPOTEN

enalapril / VASOTEC

lisinopril / PRINIVIL, ZESTRIL

quinapril / ACCUPRIL

moexipril / UNIVASC

Interactions

Food: Food can decrease the absorption of captopril and moexipril. So take captopril and moexipril one hour before or two hours after meals. ACE inhibitors may increase the amount of potassium in your body. Too much potassium can be harmful. Make sure to tell your doctor if you are taking potassium supplements or diuretics (water pills) that may increase the amount of potassium in your body. Avoid eating large amounts of foods high in potassium such as bananas, green leafy vegetables, and oranges.

HMG-CoA Reductase Inhibitors/Statins

These medications are used to lower cholesterol. They work to reduce the rate of production of LDL (bad cholesterol). Some of these drugs also lower triglycerides. Recent studies have shown that pravastatin can reduce the risk of heart attack, stroke, or miniature stroke in certain patient populations.

Some examples are:

atorvastatin / LIPITOR

fluvastatin / LESCOL

lovastatin / MEVACOR

pravastatin / PRAVACHOL

simvastatin / ZOCOR

Alcohol: Avoid drinking large amounts of alcohol because it may increase the risk of liver damage.

Food: Lovastatin (Mevacor) should be taken with the evening meal to enhance effectiveness. Grapefruit, grapefruit juice, and certain citrus fruits should be avoided with statins due to the potential for increased drug toxicity.

Anticoagulants

Anticoagulants help to prevent the formation of blood clots.

An example is:

warfarin / COUMADIN

Interactions

Food: Vitamin K produces blood-clotting substances and may reduce the effectiveness of anticoagulants. So limit the amount of foods high in vitamin K (such as broccoli, spinach, kale, turnip greens, cauliflower, and brussels sprouts) and keep vitamin K intake consistent. High doses of vitamin E (400 IU or more) may prolong clotting time and increase the risk of bleeding. Talk to your doctor before taking vitamin E supplements.

Infections

Antibiotics and Antifungals

Many different types of drugs are used to treat infections caused by bacteria and fungi. Some general advice to follow when taking any such product is:

- Tell your doctor about any skin rashes you may have had with antibiotics or that you get while taking this medication. A rash can be a symptom of an allergic reaction, and allergic reactions can be very serious.
- Tell your doctor if you experience diarrhea.
- If you are using birth control, consult with your healthcare provider because some methods may not work when taken with antibiotics.
- Be sure to finish all your medication even if you are feeling better.
- Take with plenty of water.

Antibiotics

Penicillin

Some examples are:

penicillin V / VEETIDS
amoxicillin / TRIMOX, AMOXIL
ampicillin / PRINCIPEN, OMNIPEN

Interaction

Food: Take on an empty stomach, but if it upsets your stomach, take it with food.

Quinolones

Some examples are:
    ciprofloxacin / CIPRO
    levofloxacin / LEVAQUIN
    ofloxacin / FLOXIN
    Interactions
Food: Take on an empty stomach one hour before or two hours after meals. If your stomach gets upset, take it with food. However, avoid calcium-containing products like milk, yogurt, vitamins or minerals containing iron, and antacids because they significantly decrease drug concentration.

Caffeine: Taking these medications with caffeine-containing products (for example, coffee, colas, tea, and chocolate) may increase caffeine levels, leading to excitability and nervousness.

Cephalosporins

Some examples are:
    cefaclor / CECLOR, CECLOR CD
    cefadroxil / DURICEF
    cefixime / SUPRAX
    cefprozil / CEFZIL
    cephalexin / KEFLEX, KEFTAB
    Interaction
Food: Take on an empty stomach one hour before or two hours after meals. If your stomach gets upset, take with food.

Macrolides

Some examples are:
    azithromycin / ZITHROMAX
    clarithromycin / BIAXIN
    erythromycin / E-MYCIN, ERY-TAB, ERYC
    erythromycin _ sulfisoxazole / PEDIAZOLE
    Interaction
Food: Take on an empty stomach one hour before or two hours after meals. If your stomach gets upset, take with food.

Sulfonamides

An example is:
    sulfamethoxazole _ trimethoprim / BACTRIM, SEPTRA

Interaction

Food: Take on an empty stomach one hour before or two hours after meals. If your stomach gets upset, take with food.

Tetracyclines

Some examples are:

tetracycline / ACHROMYCIN, SUMYCIN
doxycycline / VIBRAMYCIN
minocycline / MINOCIN

Interaction

Food: Take on an empty stomach one hour before or two hours after meals. If your stomach gets upset, take with food. However, it is important to avoid taking tetracycline / ACHROMYCIN, SUMYCIN with dairy products, antacids, and vitamins containing iron because these can interfere with the medication's effectiveness.

Nitroimidazole

An example is:

metronidazole / FLAGYL

Interaction

Alcohol: Avoid drinking alcohol or using medications that contain alcohol or eating foods prepared with alcohol while you are taking metronidazole and for at least three days after you finish the medication. Alcohol may cause nausea, abdominal cramps, vomiting, headaches, and flushing.

Antifungals

Some examples are:

fluconazole / DIFLUCAN
griseofulvin / GRIFULVIN
ketoconazole / NIZORAL
itraconazole / SPORANOX
terbinafine / LAMISIL

Interactions

Food: It is important to avoid taking these medications with dairy products (milk, cheeses, yogurt, ice cream) or antacids.

Alcohol: Avoid drinking alcohol, using medications that contain alcohol, or eating foods prepared with alcohol while you are taking ketoconazole/NIZORAL and for at least three days after you finish the medication. Alcohol may cause nausea, abdominal cramps, vomiting, headaches, and flushing.

Mood Disorders

Depression, Emotional, and Anxiety Disorders

Depression, panic disorder, and anxiety are a few examples of mood disorders—complex medical conditions with varying degrees of severity. When using medications to treat mood disorders it is important to follow your doctor's instructions. Remember to take your dose as directed even if you are feeling better, and do not stop unless you consult your doctor. In some cases it may take several weeks to see an improvement in symptoms.

Monoamine Oxidase (MAO) Inhibitors

Some examples are:
   phenelzine / NARDIL
   tranylcypromine / PARNATE
   Interactions
MAO Inhibitors have many dietary restrictions, and people taking them need to follow the dietary guidelines and physician's instructions very carefully. A rapid, potentially fatal increase in blood pressure can occur if foods or alcoholic beverages containing tyramine are consumed while taking MAO Inhibitors.

   Alcohol: Do not drink beer, red wine, other alcoholic beverages, non-alcoholic and reduced-alcohol beer, and red wine products.

   Food: Foods high in tyramine that should be avoided include:

- American processed; cheddar, blue, brie, mozzarella, and Parmesan cheese; yogurt, sour cream.
- Beef or chicken liver; cured meats such as sausage and salami; game meat; caviar; dried fish.
- Avocados, bananas, yeast extracts, raisins, sauerkraut, soy sauce, miso soup.
- Broad (fava) beans, ginseng, caffeine-containing products (colas, chocolate, coffee, and tea).

Anti-Anxiety Drugs

Some examples are:
    lorazepam / ATIVAN
    diazepam / VALIUM
    alprazolam / XANAX
    Interactions
    Alcohol: May impair mental and motor performance (e.g., driving, operating machinery).

    Caffeine: May cause excitability, nervousness, and hyperactivity and lessen the anti-anxiety effects of the drugs.

Antidepressant Drugs

Some examples are:
    paroxetine / PAXIL
    sertraline / ZOLOFT
    fluoxetine / PROZAC
    citalopram / CELEXA
    Interactions
    Alcohol: Although alcohol may not significantly interact with these drugs to affect mental or motor skills, people who are depressed should not drink alcohol.

    Food: These medications can be taken with or without food.

Stomach Conditions

Conditions like acid reflux, heartburn, acid indigestion, sour stomach, and gas are very common ailments. The goal of treatment is to relieve pain, promote healing, and prevent the irritation from returning. This is achieved by either reducing the acid the body creates or protecting the stomach from the acid. Lifestyle and dietary habits can play a large role in the symptoms of these conditions. For example, smoking cigarettes and consuming products that contain caffeine may make symptoms return.

Histamine Blockers

Some examples are:
    cimetidine / TAGAMET or TAGAMET HB

famotidine / PEPCID or PEPCID AC
ranitidine / ZANTAC or ZANTAC 75
nizatadine / AXID or AXID AR
Interactions

Alcohol: Avoid alcohol while taking these products. Alcohol may irritate the stomach and make it more difficult for the stomach to heal.

Food: Can be taken with or without regard to meals.

Caffeine: Caffeine products (for example, cola, chocolate, tea, and coffee) may irritate the stomach.

Drug-to-Drug Interactions

Not only can drugs interact with food and alcohol, they can also interact with each other. Some drugs are given together on purpose for an added effect, like codeine and acetaminophen for pain relief. But other drug-to-drug interactions may be unintended and harmful. Prescription drugs can interact with each other or with over-the-counter (OTC) drugs, such as acetaminophen, aspirin, and cold medicine.

Likewise, OTC drugs can interact with each other.

Sometimes the effect of one drug may be increased or decreased. For example, tricyclic antidepressants such as amitriptyline (ELAVIL), or nortriptyline (PAMELOR) can decrease the ability of clonidine (CATAPRES) to lower blood pressure. In other cases, the effects of a drug can increase the risk of serious side effects. For example, some antifungal medications such as itraconazole (SPORANOX) and ketoconazole (NIZORAL) can interfere with the way some cholesterol-lowering medications are broken down by the body. This can increase the risk of a serious side effect.

Doctors can often prescribe other medications to reduce the risk of drug-to-drug interactions. For example, two cholesterol-lowering drugs—pravastatin (PRAVACHOL) and fluvastatin (LESCOL)—are less likely to interact with antifungal medications. Be sure to tell your doctor about all medications—prescription and OTC—that you are taking.

Source: The National Consumers League 2004.

A10. INSULIN ACTION TIMES

Activity of Insulin Preparations

Type of Insulin	Examples	Onset of Action	Peak of Action	Duration of Action
Rapid-Acting	Humalog (lispro) Eli Lilly	15 minutes	30–90 minutes	3–5 hours
	NovoLog (aspart) Novo Nordisk	15 minutes	40–50 minutes	3–5 hours
Short-Acting (Regular)	Humulin R Eli Lilly Novolin R Novo Nordisk	30–60 minutes	50–120 minutes	5–8 hours
Intermediate-Acting (NPH)	Humulin N Eli Lilly Novolin N Novo Nordisk	1–3 hours	8 hours	20 hours
	Humulin L Eli Lilly Novolin L Novo Nordisk	1–2.5 hours	7–15 hours	18–24 hours
Intermediate- and Short-Acting Mixtures	Humulin 50/50 Humulin 70/30 Humalog Mix 75/25 Humalog Mix 50/50 Eli Lilly Novolin 70/30 NovoLog Mix 70/30 Novo Nordisk			
	The onset, peak, and duration of action for these mixtures would reflect a composite of the intermediate-, short-, or rapid-acting components with one peak of action.			

(continues)

(Continued)

Type of Insulin	Examples	Onset of Action	Peak of Action	Duration of Action
Long-Acting	Ultralente Eli Lilly	4–8 hours	8–12 hours	36 hours
	Lantus (glargine) Aventis	1 hour	none	24 hours

Source: Food and Drug Administration, http://www.fda.gov.

A11. MEDICAL TERMINOLOGY

Acronym	Term	More Information
ABG	arterial blood gases	A type of test measuring oxygen and carbon dioxide in the blood to detect lung function.
ACE	angiotensin converting enzyme	A class of drugs used to treat high blood pressure, heart failure, diabetes, and kidney diseases.
ACL	anterior cruciate ligament	The most important of the four major ligaments connecting the knee to the bone.
ADHD	attention deficit hyperactivity disorder	A neurobehaviorial development disorder characterized by difficulty to stay focused and control self-behavior, and overactivity.
AFIB	atrial fibrillation	A disturbance of the rhythm of the heart (*also,* A Fib).
AIDS	acquired immunodeficiency syndrome (AIDS)	Infection caused by human immunodeficiency virus (HIV)
ALP	alkaline phosphatase	A group of enzymes found in the liver and bone; a test for ALP helps to detect liver disease or bone disorders.
ALS	amyotrophic lateral sclerosis	A disease of the nerves in the brain and spinal cord that determine voluntary movement (*also,* Lou Gehrig's disease).
ALT	alanine aminotransferase	A type of enzyme; a blood test for ALP can detect liver disease.
AMD	age-related macular degeneration	A disease in older adults that causes loss of sharp, central vision.

(Continued)

Acronym	Term	More Information
AMI	acute myocardial infarction	Interruption of blood to a part of the heart (*also*, heart attack).
AODM	adult onset diabetes mellitus	Type 2 diabetes (formerly non-insulin-dependent diabetes melllitus, NIDDM). A mild form of diabetes found in adults after age 45, resulting from obesity or severe stress.
AST	aspartate aminotransferase	An enzyme found in blood cells, heart, muscle tissue, liver, pancreas, and kidneys. A blood test for ALP can detect organ damage or liver disease.
AVM	arteriovenous malformation	A defect in the circulatory system.
BID	twice a day	Note about frequency of a medication or therapy on prescriptions and medical charts.
BMI	body mass index	A measure of body fat based on weight and height.
BP	blood pressure	The force of blood pushing against arterial walls.
BPH	benign prostatic hypertrophy	Enlargement of the prostate gland; can mimic cancer.
BRCA		A type of breast gene linked to an increased risk for breast or ovarian cancer.
BUN	blood urea nitrogen	A type of test measuring the amount of nitrogen in the waste product urea; used to detect kidney abnormalities and disease.
CA	cancer	The uncontrolled growth of abnormal cells in the body.
Ca	calcium	An element. A blood test used to determine the amount of Ca not in bones.
CA-125	cancer antigen 125	A type of blood test used to measure cancer activity.
CABG	coronary artery bypass graft	A type of surgery used to increase blood flow to the heart.
CAD	coronary artery disease	A narrowing of the small blood vessels supplying oxygen and blood to the heart.

(continues)

(Continued)

Acronym	Term	More Information
CAT	computerized axial tomography	A type of diagnostic imager using a series of x-ray scans and data analysis to detect organ structure.
CBC	complete blood count	A type of test that measures the number of red and white blood cells, amount of hemoglobin, and percent of hematocrit in red blood cells.
CHD	congenital heart disease	Inherited disease of the heart.
CHF	congestive heart failure	A condition in which the heart can't pump enough blood throughout the body (*also,* heart failure).
CMV	cytomegalovirus	A species of virus that infects most humans at some time in their life but does not cause an obvious illness (e.g., herpes simplex).
CNS	central nervous system	The part of the nervous system comprising the brain and spinal cord.
COPD	chronic obstructive pulmonary disease	A progressive disease that makes it hard to breathe.
CPK	creatine phosphokinase	An enzyme found in the heart, brain, and skeleton. A blood test for CPK helps determine muscle injury to the heart.
CPR	cardiopulmonary resuscitation	A rescue emergency procedure used when the heart has stopped or the person is no longer breathing.
CRF	chronic renal failure	Failure of the kidneys to function properly.
CRP	C-reactive protein	A type of protein found in the blood; levels rise with inflammation or heart problems.
CSF	cerebrospinal fluid	A colorless, protective, and nourishing liquid that surrounds the brain and spinal cord.
CVA	cerebrovascular accident	An interruption of the blood supply to the brain (*also,* stroke, brain attack).
CXR	chest x-ray	A type of diagnostic test using radiation to image abnormalities of the lungs, heart, or bones.
D&C	dilatation and curettage	A surgical procedure enlarging and scraping the lining of the uterus (womb).

(Continued)

Acronym	Term	More Information
DJD	degenerative joint disease	A progressive stiffness and pain in the joints (*also,* arthritis).
DM	diabetes mellitus	A group of metabolic disorders characterized by high blood sugar levels due to defects of insulin production.
DTP	diphtheria, tetanus, pertussis	A type of vaccine to immunize against three infectious diseases.
DVT	deep-vein thrombosis	A blood clot in the large vein of the lower legs.
DX	diagnosis	A notation in a medical chart.
ECG, EKG	electrocardiogram	A noninvasive test that measures electrical impulses of the heart.
ECHO	echocardiogram	A sonogram test that uses sound waves to image the heart.
EEG	electroencephalogram	A test that measures electrical impulses of the brain.
EMG	electromyography	A test that measures electrical impulses of muscles.
ENT	ear, nose and throat	A branch of medicine (*also,* otolaryngology).
ERCP	endoscopic retrograde cholangiopancreatography	A procedure using a small lighted instrument to diagnose problems in the liver, gallbladder, bile ducts, and pancreas.
ESR	erythrocyte sedimentation rate	A test measuring how quickly red blood cells settle in a test tube after one hour; used to detect inflammation.
ESRD	end-stage renal disease	The complete or almost complete failure of the kidneys to function.
FSH	follicle stimulating hormone	A hormone produced by the pituitary gland; controls production of eggs in women and sperm in men; a test to evaluate fertility.
GERD	gastroesophageal reflux disease	A progressive condition where the stomach contents leak backwards into your gullet (also, acid reflux, heartburn).
GI	gastrointestinal	Digestive system from the mouth to the anus.

(continues)

(Continued)

Acronym	Term	More Information
GFR	glomerular filtration rate	A measure of how much blood passes through the tiny tubular filters in the kidney; tests kidney function.
GU	genitourinary	Organ system of the urinary and reproductive organs.
HAV	hepatitis A virus	A Picornavirus that causes inflammation of the liver.
HBV	hepatitis B virus	A family Orthohepadadnavirus that infects the liver; transmitted via sexual intercourse, IV drug use, or exposure to infected blood.
HCT	hematocrit	A type of test to measure the number of red blood cells in the blood.
HCV	hepatitis C virus	A family Flavivirdae virus transmitted via blood-to-blood contact that causes damage to the liver.
HDL	high density lipoprotein	Smallest and densest of the lipoproteins synthesized in the liver; captures and transports cholesterol from the bloodstream to the liver for excretion (*also*, good cholesterol).
HGB	hemoglobin	A protein in red blood cells that carries oxygen.
HIV	human immunodeficiency virus	A lentivirus of the Retrovirus family; gradually destroys the immune system.
HPV	human papillomavirus	A member of the Papilloma family of viruses that infects humans by sexual transmission. Most do not know they are infected, and 90% will naturally become immune within two years. Can cause genital and throat warts and cervical and penile cancers (*also*, genital human papillomavirus).
HRT	hormone replacement therapy	Medications to replace the female hormones no longer naturally made during and after menopause.
HTN	hypertension	High blood pressure.
IBD	inflammatory bowel disease	A group of inflammatory conditions of the colon and small intestine; primarily ulcerative colitis and Crohn's disease.

(Continued)

Acronym	Term	More Information
IBS	irritable bowel syndrome	A disorder involving cramping, abdominal pain, and bowel movement changes; involves the large intestine.
ICD	implantable cardioverter defibrillator	A small device that uses electrical impulses to control heart rhythm in patients with life-threatening irregular heartbeats.
ICU	intensive care unit	A facility in a hospital where critically ill patients are treated by specially-trained healthcare staff.
IDDM	insulin-dependent diabetes mellitus	Former name for type 1 diabetes; typically discovered in childhood when the body produces insufficient or no insulin to manage blood glucose levels (*also,* juvenile diabetes).
IM	intramuscular	A type of needle injection of a fluid into the muscle.
IUD	intrauterine device	A small plastic device inserted into the uterus as a method of birth control.
IV	intravenous	A type of needle injection of a medication into the blood vessel (IV).
IVP	intravenous pyelogram	An x-ray test of the kidneys, bladder, and ureters.
LDL	low density lipoprotein	A type of lipoprotein that delivers cholesterol to the body; high levels indicate cardiovascular disease (*also,* bad cholesterol).
LFT	liver function tests	A group of tests that together evaluate liver damage.
MI	myocardial infarction	When the heart muscle tissue dies or loses function because of a lack of oxygen from blocked blood vessels to the heart (*also,* heart attack).
MMR	measles, mumps, and rubella	A vaccine to immunize against three diseases.
MRI	magnetic resonance imaging	A device that uses magnetism and radio wave energy to visualize and record organs and structures inside of the body; scans can be in layers.

(continues)

(Continued)

Acronym	Term	More Information
MRSA	methicillin-resistant *Staphylococcus aureus*	A bacterial infection that is highly resistant to antibiotics.
MS	multiple sclerosis	An autoimmune disease that affects the central nervous system; damages the myelin sheath around the nerves, causing them to slow or stop firing.
NG	nasogastric	Passage from the nose to the stomach.
NIDDM	non-insulin-dependent diabetes mellitus	Former name for type 2 diabetes; chronic disease marked by high levels of glucose in the blood; appears generally around age 45 (*also,* adult-onset diabetes).
NKDA	no known drug allergies	A type of notation in a medical history chart.
NSAID	non-steroidal anti-inflammatory drug	Commonly prescribed drugs for inflammation and pain.
OCD	obsessive-compulsive disorder	A type of anxiety disorder where people have unwanted, intrusive thoughts causing apprehension and/or repetitive behaviors performed in the hopes of calming themselves.
PAD	peripheral arterial disease	Diseases of the arteries outside of the heart; can refer to plaque buildup in the arteries.
PAP	Papanicolau	A type of screening test used to detect abnormal cervical or cancerous cells in the uterus (*also,* Pap smear, cervical test, smear test).
PAT	paroxysmal atrial tachycardia	A disturbance of the rhythm of the heart where it beats very rapidly and regularly before stopping abruptly.
PET	positron emission tomography	A type of imaging test using nuclear medicine tracer to create a three-dimensional picture of the organs.
PFT	pulmonary function test	A type of test to measure lung function.
PID	pelvic inflammatory disease	A type of sexually transmitted infection of the female reproductive organs.
PMS	premenstrual syndrome	A group of symptoms that may happen 5–10 days before menstruation and stops when menstruation occurs.

(Continued)

Acronym	Term	More Information
PPD	purified protein derivative	An extract of Mycobacterium tuberculosis injected under the skin to test for an immune response to tuberculosis.
PRN	as needed	A notation often made in medical notes and prescriptions to signify the frequency to take a medication or therapy.
PSA	prostate specific antigen	A type of screening test to detect prostate cancer.
PT	prothrombin time	A test to measure the time it takes for liquid portion of blood (plasma) to clot; used to monitor bleeding difficulties, Vitamin K deficiency, and liver disease.
PTH	parathyroid hormone	A polypeptide that regulates calcium and phosphorus concentrations in extracellular fluid; used to test for parathyroid disease and hyperparathyroidism.
PTSD	post-traumatic stress syndrome	A severe anxiety disorder that occurs after a traumatic event (e.g., military combat, violent personal assaults, natural or human disasters, etc.).
PTT	partial thromboplastin time	A blood test to measure clotting time used to determine the cause of abnormal bleeding or bruising, check levels of clotting factors, and check for conditions affecting clotting.
PUD	peptic ulcer disease	Sores or eroded areas lining the gastrointestinal tract, primarily the stomach; caused by the bacteria *Helicobacter pylori* or NSAIDS.
PVC	premature ventricular contraction	A disturbance of the rhythm of the heart involving irregular or skipped heartbeats.
QID	four times a day	A type of notation written in a prescription or medical record.
RA	rheumatoid arthritis	An autoimmune disease causing long-term inflammation in the joints and eventually the surrounding tissues and organs.

(continues)

(Continued)

Acronym	Term	More Information
RBC	red blood cell	A type of cell in the bloodstream that delivers oxygen and removes waste from other cells and tissues in the body (*also*, erythrocyte).
RSV	respiratory syncytial virus	A virus that causes infections in the lungs and respiratory tract of children and adults; symptoms are mild in most people, and typically mimic the common cold.
Rx	treatment	A notation on a medical record or prescription.
SAD	seasonal affective disorder	A mood disorder where episodes of depression occur during the fall and winter months that disappear with spring and summer; some respond to full spectrum light therapy and antidepressants (*also*, winter blues).
SIDS	sudden infant death syndrome	The unexpected death of a child under 1 year of age where there are no symptoms or definable cause.
SLE	systemic lupus erythematosus	A chronic or acute autoimmune disorder that affects various body tissues, where an overactive immune system attacks healthy cells (*also*, lupus).
SOB	shortness of breath	Gasping for air that is not explained by rigorous exercise or exertion (*also*, dyspepnia).
STD	sexually transmitted disease	A type of infection that occurs after having sex with an infected person; includes Chlamydia, syphilis, gonorrhea, herpes, HIV, and genital warts (*also*, venereal disease [VD], sexually transmitted infection [STI]).
T3	triiodothyronine	One of the thyroid hormones used to detect thyroid disease.
T4	thyroxine	An iodine-producing hormone found in the thyroid; used to treat or prevent goiter and other thyroid disorders.
TB	tuberculosis	A contagious bacterial infection that affects primarily the lungs but may spread to other organs.

(Continued)

Acronym	Term	More Information
TAH	total abdominal hysterectomy	Surgery to remove a woman's uterus (womb).
TIA	transient ischemic attack	An episode of brief stroke-like symptoms lasting for 1–2 hours; a warning sign of an impending stroke.
TIBC	total iron binding capacity	A test to measure the amount of iron in the blood.
TID	three times a day	A notation about how often to take a drug or therapy on a medical chart or prescription.
TMJ	temporomandibular joint	The joint that connects your jaw to the side of your head.
TORCH	toxoplasmosis, rubella, cytomegalovirus, herpes simplex, and HIV	A blood screening test for a group of infections that may cause birth defects; administered to newborns and sometimes their mothers.
TSH	thyroid stimulating hormone	A hormone produced by the pituitary gland that regulates the thyroid. A blood test for TSH can detect abnormal thyroid function.
TURP	transurethral resection of prostate gland	Surgery to remove parts of the prostate gland.
URI	upper respiratory infection	Bacterial or viral infection in the respiratory tract; ranges from the common cold to life-threatening illnesses such as epiglottitis.
UTI	urinary tract infection	An infection that most often begins in the bladder or urethra, but also can be in the ureters or kidneys.
XRT	radiotherapy	External beam radiation therapy; uses radiation to treat localized cancer (*also*, X-ray therapy).
WBC	white blood cell	One of the cells in the body's immune system that helps fight infection (*also*, leukocyte).

Source: MedlinePlus, a service of the U.S. National Library of Medicine and National Institutes of Health. Available at: http://www.nlm.nih.gov/medlineplus/appendixb.html

REFERENCES

1. Shah B, Sucher K, Hollenbeck C. Comparison of ideal body weight equations and published height-weight tables with body mass index tables for healthy adults in the United States. *Nutr Clin Pract.* 2006; 21:312.

2. Delegge MH, Drake LM. Nutritional assessment. *Gastroenterol Clin N Am.* 2007; 36:1–22.

3. Mifflin MD, St Jeor ST, Hill LA, Scott BJ, Daugherty SA, Koh YO. A new predictive equation for resting energy expenditure in healthy individuals. *Am J Clin Nutr.* 1990; 51(2):241–247.

4. World Health Organization (WHO). Energy and protein requirements. (1991). Accessed April 5, 2011 from http://www.fao.org/docrep/003/aa040e/AA040E06 .htm

5. Anastasio C, Nagel R. Home enteral nutrition in the pediatric patient. In: Ireton-Jones CS, DeLegge MH, eds. *Handbook of Home Nutrition Support.* Sudbury, MA: Jones and Bartlett Publishers; 2007: 153–222.

6. Curreri PW, Richmond D, Marvin J, Baxter CR. Classic article: dietary requirements of patients with major burns. *Nutr Clin Pract.* 2001; 16;169–171.

7. Dickerson R, Gervasio J, Riley M, et al. Accuracy of predictive methods to estimate resting energy expenditure of thermally-injured patients. *J Parenter Enteral Nutr.* 2002; 26:17–29.

8. Ireton-Jones C, Jones JD. Improved equations for predicting energy expenditure in patients: the Ireton-Jones equations. *Nutr Clin Pract.* 2002; 17:29–31.

9. McClave SA, Robert G. Martindale RG, et al. Guidelines for the provision and assessment of nutrition support therapy in the adult critically ill patient: Society of Critical Care Medicine (SCCM) and American Society for Parenteral and Enteral Nutrition (A.S.P.E.N.). *J Parenter Enteral Nutr.* 2009; 33(3):277–316.

Selected Formula

ADULT AND PEDIATRIC ORAL
AND ENTERAL FORMULAS

Partial Listing of Enteral Formulas

Sample Standard Fiber-Free Formulas, Selected Nutrient Data

	Nutren® 1.0 (Nestlé)	Osmolite® 1 CAL (Abbott)	Isosource® HN (Nestlé)	Osmolite® 1.2 CAL (Abbott)	Nutren® 1.5 (Nestlé)	Osmolite® 1.5 CAL (Abbott)
Serving Size	1000 mL	1000 mL	1000 mL	1000 mL	1000 mL	1000 mL
Calories	1000	1060	1200	1200	1,500	1500
Protein (g)	40	44.3	53	55.5	60	62.7
Fat (g)	38	34.7	39	39.3	67.6	49.1
Carbohydrate (g)	127	143.9	160	157.5	169	203.6
Water (mL)	848	842	818	820	775	762
Vitamin A (IU)	3200	3790	4300	5000	4800	8320
Vitamin D (IU)	267	305	340	400	400	400
Vitamin K (µg)	50	61	80	80	75	80
Vitamin C (mg)	140	230	200	300	212	240
Sodium (mg)	876	930	1100	1340	1168	1400
Potassium (mg)	1248	1570	1900	1810	1872	1800
Calcium (mg)	668	760	1200	1200	1000	1000
Phosphorus (mg)	668	760	1200	1200	1000	1000
Zinc (mg)	14	18	19	23	20	23
Magnesium (mg)	268	305	350	400	400	400
Iron (mg)	12	14	15	18	18	18
Osmolality (mOsm/kg)	370	300	490	360	430	525
Volume for 100% RDI (mL)	1500	1321	1165	1000	1000	1000

Sample Standard with Fiber Formulas, Selected Nutrient Data

	Jevity® 1 CAL (Abbott)	Nutren®1.0 Fiber (Nestlé)	Jevity® 1.2 CAL (Abbott)	Fibersource HN® (Nestlé)	Jevity® 1.5 CAL (Abbott)	Isosource® 1.5 CAL (Nestlé)	Compleat® (Nestlé)
Serving Size	1000 mL	1000 mL	1000 mL	1000 mL	1000 mL	1000 mL	1000 mL
Calories	1060	1000	1200	1200	1500	1500	1070
Protein (g)	44.3	40	55.5	53	63.8	68	48
Fat (g)	34.7	38	39.3	39	49.8	65	40
Carbohydrate (g)	154.7	127	169.4	160	215.7	170	128
Dietary Fiber (g)	14.4	14	18.0	10.0	22.0	8.0	6.0
Water (mL)	835	838	807	810	760	778	854
Vitamin A (IU)	3790	3200	5000	4300	5000	10700	3800
Vitamin D (IU)	305	267	400	340	400	430	300
Vitamin K (µg)	61	50	80	80	80	86	61
Vitamin C (mg)	230	140	300	200	300	320	46
Sodium (mg)	930	876	1350	1200	1400	1290	1000
Potassium (mg)	1570	1248	1850	2000	2150	2250	1720
Calcium (mg)	910	668	1200	1000	1200	1070	760
Phosphorus (mg)	760	668	1200	1000	1200	1070	760
Zinc (mg)	18	14	23	19	23	32	11
Magnesium (mg)	305	268	400	350	400	430	300
Iron (mg)	14	12	18	17	18	19	14
Osmolality (mOsm/kg)	300	410	450	490	525	650	340
Volume for 100% RDI (mL)	1321	1500	1000	1165	1000	933	1313

Sample Critical Care/Healing Support Formulas, Selected Nutrient Data

	Nutren® Replete® (Nestlé)	Promote® (Abbott)	Nutren® Replete® Fiber (Nestlé)	Promote® with Fiber (Abbott)	Perative® (Abbott)	Crucial® (Nestlé)	Pivot® 1.5 CAL (Abbott)	Peptamen® Bariatric (Nestlé)	Impact® (Nestlé)	Impact® with Fiber (Nestlé)	Impact® Glutamine (Nestlé)	Oxepa® (Abbott)	Impact® Peptide 1.5 (Nestlé)
Serving Size	1000 mL	1000 mL	1000 mL	1000 mL	1000 mL	1000 mL	1000 mL	1000 mL	1000 mL	1000 mL	1000 mL	1000 mL	1000 mL
Calories	1000	1000	1000	1000	1300	1500	1500	1000	1000	1000	1300	1500	1500
Protein (g)	62.4	62.5	62.4	62.5	66.7	94	93.8	93.3	56	56	78	62.7	94
Fat (g)	34	26.0	34	28.2	37.3	67.6	50.8	38	28	28	43	93.8	63.6
Carbohydrate (g)	113	130	113	138.3	180.3	134	172.4	77.8	130	140	150	105.3	140
Dietary Fiber (g)	–	–	14	14.4	6.5	–	7.5	4.3	–	10	10	–	–
Water (mL)	845	839	835	831	790	772	759	840	853	868	808	785	770
Vitamin A (IU)	5000	7250	5000	7250	8675	15000	10000	6670	6700	6700	8700	11910	15000
Vitamin D (IU)	272	400	272	400	350	400	400	280	270	270	400	425	400
Vitamin E	60	45	60	45	40	100	250	100	60	60	78	85	100
Vitamin K (µg)	50	80	50	80	70	75	80	50	67	67	80	850	75
Vitamin C (mg)	340	345	340	340	260	1000	300	320	80	80	260	1310	1000
Sodium (mg)	876	1000	876	1300	1040	1168	1400	670	1100	1100	1320	1960	1170
Potassium (mg)	1500	1980	1500	2100	1735	1872	2000	1330	1760	1820	2160	1060	1870

(continues)

(Continued)

Calcium (mg)	1000	1200	1000	1200	870	1000	1000	670	800	800	1200	1060	1000
Phosphorus (mg)	1000	1200	1000	1200	870	1000	1000	670	800	800	1200	425	1000
Magnesium (mg)	400	400	400	400	350	400	400	267	270	270	400	24	420
Zinc (mg)	24	24	24	24	20	36	25	24	15	15	20	20	36
Iron (mg)	18	18	18	18	16.0	18	18	12	12	12	18	535	18
Osmolality (mOsm/kg)	300	340	310	380	460	490	595	345	375	375	630	946	510
Volume for 100% RDI (mL)	1000	1000	1000	1000	1155	1000	1000	1500	1500	1500	1000		1000

Sample Elemental and Semi-Elemental Formulas, Selected Nutrient Data*

	Peptamen® (Nestlé)	Vital® 1.0 CAL(Abbott)	Peptamen® 1.5 (Nestlé)	Vital® 1.5 CAL(Abbott)	Optimental® (Abbott)	Vital® HN (Abbott)	Vivonex® Plus (Nestlé)	Vivonex® RTF (Nestlé)	Vivonex® T.E.N (Nestlé)
Serving Size	1000 mL	1000 mL	1000 mL	1000 mL	1000 mL	1000 mL	1000 mL	1000 mL	1000 mL
Calories	1000	1000	1500	1500	1000	1000	1000	1000	1000
Protein (g)	40	40	67.6	67.5	51.3	41.7	45	50	38
Fat (g)	39	38.1	56	57.1	28.4	10.8	6.7	12	2.8
Carbohydrate (g)	127	130	188	187	139	185.0	190	175	210
Dietary Fiber (g)	—	4.2	—	6.0	5.0	—	—	—	—
Water (mL)	848	842	771	764	832	867	825	848	825
Vitamin A (IU)	4300	4570	6460	6500	8290	3332	2780	3300	2500
Vitamin D (IU)	272	280	408	400	285	267	220	270	200
Vitamin K (µg)	50	56	75	80	85	54	44	53	40
Vitamin C (mg)	340	350	512	500	215	200	67	67	60
Sodium (mg)	560	1055	1020	1500	1125	566	610	670	600
Potassium (mg)	1500	1400	1860	2000	1705	1400	1060	1200	950
Calcium (mg)	800	705	1000	1000	1055	667	560	670	500
Phosphorus (mg)	700	705	1000	1000	1055	667	560	670	500
Magnesium (mg)	300	280	400	400	425	267	220	270	200
Zinc (mg)	24	21	36	30	16	15	13	13	11
Iron (mg)	18	13	27	18	13	12	10	12	9.0
Osmolality (mOsm/kg)	270	390	550	610	585	500	650	630	630
Volume for 100% RDI (mL)	1500	1422	1000	1000	1422	1500	1800	1500	2000

*See also Critical Care and Healing Support table; the following formulas are also semi-elemental according to manufacturer information: Crucial®, Impact Glutamine®, Pivot®, and Perative®.

Sample Renal Formulas, Selected Nutrient Data

	Nepro® with Carb Steady® (Abbott)	Suplena® with Carb Steady® (Abbott)*	Renalcal® (Nestlé)	Nova source® Renal (Nestlé)
Serving Size	1000 mL	1000 mL	1000 mL	1000 mL
Calories	1800	1795	2000	2000
Protein (g)	81	45	34.4	90.7
Fat (g)	96	96	82.4	100
Carbohydrate (g)	161	196	290.4	183
Dietary Fiber (g)	12.6	12.7	—	—
Water (mL)	727	738	700	717
Vitamin A (IU)	3180	3165	—	3000
Vitamin D (IU)	85	84	—	400
Vitamin K (µg)	85	84	—	80
Folic Acid(µg)	1060	1055	600	1000
Vitamin C (mg)	105	106	60	60
Sodium (mg)	1060	802	—	945
Potassium (mg)	1060	1139	—	945
Calcium (mg)	1060	1055	—	840
Phosphorus (mg)	720	717	—	819
Magnesium (mg)	210	211	—	197
Zinc (mg)	27	27	14	22
Iron (mg)	19	19	—	18
Osmolality (mOsm/kg)	745	780	600	800
Volume for 100% RDI (mL)	944	944	1000	1000

*1000 mL values calculated as 1L container is not available.

Sample Diabetes Formulas, Selected Nutrient Data

	Glucerna® 1.0 CAL (Abbott)	Glucerna® 1.2 CAL (Abbott)	Glucerna® 1.5 CAL (Abbott)	Diabeti-source® AC (Nestlé)	Nutren® Glytrol® (Nestlé)
Serving Size	1000 mL	1000 mL	1000 mL	1000 mL	1000 mL
Calories	1000	1200	1500	1200	1000
Protein (g)	41.8	60	82.5	60	45.2
Fat (g)	54.4	60	75	59	47.6
Carbohydrate (g)	95.6	114.5	133.1	100	100
Dietary Fiber (g)	14.4	16.1	16.1	15	15.2
Water (mL)	853	805	759	818	840
Vitamin A (IU)	6300	7730	8660	4000	5080
Vitamin D (IU)	285	345	430	320	272
Vitamin K (µg)	57	100	125	64	50
Vitamin C (mg)	215	260	325	240	140
Sodium (mg)	930	1110	1380	1060	740
Potassium (mg)	1570	2020	2520	1720	1400
Calcium (mg)	705	800	1000	800	720
Phosphorus (mg)	705	800	1000	800	720
Magnesium (mg)	285	320	400	320	286
Zinc (mg)	16	12	15	15	15.2
Iron (mg)	13	15	18	14	12.8
Osmolality (mOsm/kg)	355	720	875	450	280
Volume for 100% RDI (mL)	1420	1250	1000	1250	1400

Sample Pulmonary Formulas, Selected Nutrient Data

	Pulmocare® (Abbott)	Nutren® Pulmonary (Nestlé)
Serving Size	1000 mL	1000 mL
Calories	1.5	1500
Protein (g)	62.6	68
Fat (g)	93.3	94.8
Carbohydrate (g)	105.7	100
Dietary Fiber (g)	—	—
Water (mL)	785	782
Vitamin A (IU)	11910	4800
Vitamin D (IU)	425	400
Vitamin K (µg)	85	74.8
Vitamin C (mg)	320	212
Sodium (mg)	1310	1168
Potassium (mg)	1960	1872
Calcium (mg)	1060	1200
Phosphorus (mg)	1060	1200
Magnesium (mg)	425	480
Zinc (mg)	24	21.2
Iron (mg)	19	18
Osmolality (mOsm/kg)	475	330
Volume for 100% RDI (mL)	947	1000

Sample Pediatric Oral and Enteral Formulas, Fiber Free, Selected Nutrient Data

Pediatric Formula Selected Nutrient Data	PediaSure® (Abbott) Standard oral	Boost® Kid Essentials 1.0 (Nestlé)	PediaSure® 1.5 (Abbott)	Boost® Kid Essentials 1.5 (Nestlé)	Nutren® Junior (Nestlé)	Peptamen® Junior (Nestlé)	Elecare® (Abbott) 30 Cal/fl oz	Vivonex® Pediatric (Nestlé)
Serving Size	1000 mL	1000 mL	8 fl oz	237 mL	1000 mL	1000 mL	1000 mL	1000 mL
Calories	1013	1000	350	355	1000	1000	1012	800
Protein (g)	30	30	14	10	30	30	30.9	24
Fat (g)	38	38	16	17.8	49.6	38.4	49	24
Carbohydrate (g)	139	135	38	39	110	138	108.6	130
Dietary Fiber (g)	4	—	—	—	—	—	—	—
L-Carnitine (mg)	17	17	4.0	6.2	40	40	—	25
Taurine (mg)	76	89	18	32	80	80	—	80
Water (mL)	844	844	185	170	852	848	842	880
Vitamin A (IU)	1688	2743	500	711	4068	4064	2769	2500
Vitamin D (IU)	506	633	160	109	560	560	607	500
Vitamin E	25	32	6.0	5.4	28	28	21.3	30
Vitamin K (μg)	68	41	16	9.5	60	30	63.9	40
Vitamin C (mg)	101	127	24	24	100	100	92	100

(continues)

(Continued)

Choline (mg)	350	422	83	95	300	300	96	200
Sodium (mg)	380	550	90	164	460	460	458	400
Potassium (mg)	1308	1140	390	309	1320	1320	1523	1200
Calcium (mg)	1055	1181	350	309	1000	1000	1172	970
Phosphorus (mg)	844	886	250	235	800	800	852	800
Magnesium (mg)	169	198	60	47	200	200	85.2	200
Zinc (mg)	6.3	12	1.5	2.8	15.2	15.2	8.5	12
Iron (mg)	11	14	2.7	3.3	14	14	14.9	10
Osmolality (mOsm/kg)	480	Vanilla: 550 Choc: 600 Strawb: 570	370	390	350	Unflavored: 260 Vanilla: 380 Choc: 380 Strawb: 400	560	360
Volume for 100% RDI (L)	Ages 1–8: 1 L Ages 9–13: 1.5 L	Ages 1–8: 1 L Ages 9–13: 1.5 L	Ages 1–8: 1 L Ages 9–13: 1.5 L	Ages 7–10: .87 L	Ages 7–10: 1000 mL	Ages 7–10: 1000	Varies	Ages 1–6: 1 L Ages 7–10: 1.17 L

Sample Pediatric Oral and Enteral Formulas, with Fiber, Selected Nutrient Data

Pediatric Formula Selected Nutrient Data	PediaSure® Enteral 1.0 with Fiber Cal (Abbott)	Nutren Junior® Fiber (Nestlé)	PediaSure® 1.5 with Fiber (Abbott)	Boost® Kid Essentials 1.5 with Fiber (Nestlé)	Compleat® Pediatric (Nestlé)	Peptamen Junior® Fiber (Nestlé)
Serving Size	1000 mL	1000 mL	8 fl oz 1	237 mL	1000 mL	1000 mL
Calories	1013	1000	350	355	1000	1000
Protein (g)	30	30	14	10	38	30
Fat (g)	38	49.6	16	17.8	39	38.4
Carbohydrate (g)	139	110	38	39	130	137
Dietary Fiber (g)	8	6	3	2.1	6.8	7.2
L-Carnitine (mg)	17	40	4.0	6.2	16	40
Taurine (mg)	76	80	18	32	84	80
Water (mL)	844	851	185	168	820	844
Vitamin A (IU)	1688	4068	500	711	3300	4072
Vitamin D (IU)	506	100	160	109	330	560
Vitamin E	25	28	6.0	5.4	21	28
Vitamin K (µg)	68	60	16	9.5	38	30
Vitamin C (mg)	101	100	24	24	96	100
Choline (mg)	350	300	83	95	500	300
Sodium (mg)	380	460	90	164	770	460
Potassium (mg)	1310	1320	390	309	1600	1320
Calcium (mg)	1055	1000	350	309	1440	1000
Phosphorus (mg)	844	800	250	235	1000	800
Magnesium (mg)	169	200	60	47	230	200
Zinc (mg)	6.3	15.2	1.5	2.8	12	15.2
Iron (mg)	11	14	2.7	3.3	13	14
Osmolality (mOsm/kg)	345	350	370	405	380	390
Volume for 100% RDI (L)	Ages 1–8: 1 L Ages 9–13:1.5 L	Ages 7–10: 1L	Ages 1–8: 1 L Ages 9–13: 1.5 L	Ages 7–10: .87 L	Ages 1–10: .9 L	Ages 7–10: 1 L

SOURCES

Abbott Nutrition. http://abbottnutrition.com/Our-Products/Our-Products.aspx Accessed November 4, 2010.

Nestlé Nutrition. http://www.nestle-nutrition.com/Products/Default.aspx Accessed November 4, 2010.

Helpful Links for the Nutrition Care Process

REFERENCE MATERIALS FOR ASSESSMENT AND MONITORING

Reference	Source(s)	Website address
Dietary Reference Intakes (DRIs) Reference values used for planning and assessing nutrient intake. Web-based tables are updated with newest DRIs as they are published.	USDA Food and Nutrition Information Center (found under Dietary Guidance heading) Food and Nutrition Board, Institute of Medicine	http://fnic.nal.usda.gov http://iom.edu/Activities/ Nutrition/SummaryDRIs/ DRI-Tables.aspx
Dietary Guidelines for Americans Evidence-based nutritional guidance to promote health and reduce chronic disease risk.	USDA	http://www.cnpp.usda.gov/ dietaryguidelines.htm

(continues)

(Continued)

Reference	Source(s)	Website address
USDA Food Composition Database View or download data on the nutrient content of over 7500 foods.	USDA	http://www.ars.usda.gov/ba/bhnrc/ndl
Growth Charts Percentile curves used to chart the growth of infants, children, and adolescents in the United States.	Center for Disease Control and Prevention	http://www.cdc.gov/growthcharts/

REFERENCE MATERIALS FOR DIAGNOSIS AND INTERVENTION

Reference	Source	Website address
ADA's Nutrition Care Process Step-by-step instructions and resources including a link for purchasing the standardized terminology manual.	American Dietetic Association Under evidence analysis library	http://www.adaevidencelibrary.com/
ADA Evidence Library Systematically reviewed scientific evidence.	American Dietetic Association Evidence Analysis library	http://www.adaevidencelibrary.com/
USDA Evidence Library Systematic reviews with supporting research for dietary guidelines.	USDA Food and Nutrition Information Center	http://fnic.nal.usda.gov

(Continued)

Reference	Source	Website address
The Cochrane Library Database of systematic reviews for healthcare decision-making.	The Cochrane Collaboration	http://www.cochrane.org/
PubMed Citations and some full-text content from biomedical literature.	The National Library of Medicine	http://www.ncbi.nlm.nih.gov/pubmed/

Abbreviations

MEASUREMENTS

L, mL, dL	liter, milliliter, deciliter
lbs	pounds
tbs/tsp	tablespoon/teaspoon
oz	ounce
mg	milligram
mEq	milliequivalent
bpm	beats per minute (heart rate)
rf	breaths per minute (respiratory rate)
h	hour (e.g., mL/h)

TERMS

5-AMA	5-aminosylicylic acid
ACS	American Cancer Society
ADA	American Dietetic Association

ADIME	A type of format to present a case defined by the *a*ssessment, *d*iagnosis, *i*ntervention, *m*onitoring, and *e*valuation
ADL	activities of daily living
AIDS	acquired immunodeficiency syndrome
BG	blood glucose
BIA	bioelectrical impedance analysis
BMI	body mass index
BPM	beats per minute
BUN	blood urea nitrogen
Ca × P	calcium times phosphorus (product)
CDC	Centers for Disease Control and Prevention
CDE	Certified Diabetes Educator
CKD	chronic kidney disease
CRF	chronic renal failure
CT	computed tomography
DRI	Dietary Reference Intakes
DV	nutritional daily value (usually in percent)
DVT	deep venous thrombosis
DXA	dual-energy X-ray absorptiometry
EEE	estimated energy requirements (EEE)
GFR	glomerular filtration rate
GI	gastrointestinal
HAART	highly active antiretroviral therapy
HbA1c	hemoglobin A1c
HDL	high density lipoprotein (cholesterol)
HIV	human immunodeficiency virus
HPT	hyperparathyroidism
Hx	history
IBD	inflammatory bowel disease
IBW	ideal body weight
ICU	intensive care unit
IDNT	International Dietetics and Nutrition Terminology

INR	international normalized ratio
IOM	Institute of Medicine
LDL	low density lipoprotein (cholesterol)
MAC	mycobacterium avium complex
MDI	multiple daily injections of insulin
MNA – SF	Mini Nutritional Assessment – Short Form
MREE	measured resting energy expenditure
MRI	magnetic resonance imaging
NPO	nothing by mouth (no eating or drinking)
NOF	National Osteoporosis Foundation
OTC	over-the-counter (medication)
PBD	post-burn day
PCOS	polycystic ovary syndrome
PEG	percutaneous endoscopic gastrostomy
PES	A statement that defines the problem related to etiology as evidenced by signs and symptoms
PRN	as needed
RD	registered dietitian
RDA	Recommended Dietary Allowances
REE	resting energy expenditure
RLQ	right lower quadrant
RQ	respiratory quotient
SMBG	self-monitoring of blood glucose
SNAP	Supplemental Nutrition Assistance Program
SOAP	Oldest type of format to assess and document nutritional care, using *s*ubjective (patient and caregiver interview and medical record; reason for the visit), *o*bjective (data from a physical exam, biochemical data, test results, etc.), *a*ssessment (brief analysis of subjective and objective data), and *p*lan (recommendations to solve the nutritional problem, including prescription, counseling/education, and/or referral to another professional).
s/p	status post
TBSA	total body surface area
TNFα	tumor necrosis factor-alpha

TPN	total parenteral nutrition
TSH	thyroid stimulating hormone
UBW	usual body weight
UC	ulcerative colitis
WHO	World Health Organization
WNL	within normal limits

Photo Credits

Chapter 1
Page 4 © Photodisc

Chapter 2
Page 10 © SuperStock/Alamy Images

Chapter 3
Page 16 © Photodisc

Chapter 4
Page 22 © Andy Lim/ShutterStock, Inc.

Chapter 5
Page 32 © Mauro Fermariello/Photo Researchers, Inc.

Chapter 6
Page 38 Courtesy of Elizabeth Platt

Chapter 10
Page 68 © crystal kirk/Fotolia.com

Chapter 11
Page 76 © forestpath/Fotolia

Chapter 12
Page 85 Courtesy of the National Institute of Diabetes and Digestive and Kidney Diseases (NIDDK)

Chapter 13
Page 92 © Don Tremain/Photodisc/Getty Images

Chapter 14
Page 98 © Djk/Dreamstime.com

Chapter 15
Page 104 © Hank Morgan/Photo Researchers, Inc.

Chapter 17
Page 122 © Andrea Danti/Fotolia.com

Chapter 18
Page 128 © sframe/Fotolia.com

Chapter 19
Page 137 © Sebastian Kaulitzki/ShutterStock, Inc.

Chapter 20
Page 144 © Bodenham, LTH NHS Trust/Photo Researchers, Inc.

Chapter 21
Page 150 Courtesy of Leonard V. Crowley, MD, Century College

Unless otherwise indicated, all photographs and illustrations are under copyright of Jones & Bartlett Learning or have been provided by the author.

Some images in this book feature models. These models do not necessarily endorse, represent, or participate in the activities represented in the images.